HEART DISEASE

HEART DISEASE

ALVIN & VIRGINIA SILVERSTEIN
& LAURA SILVERSTEIN NUNN

Twenty-First Century Medical Library

Twenty-First Century Books/Minneapolis

Cover photograph courtesy of © Tarhill Photos, Inc./CORBIS

Photographs courtesy of © CORBIS SYGMA: p. 9; National Library of Medicine/National Institutes of Health: p. 11; © Bettmann/CORBIS: pp. 15, 76; © Michel Gilles/Photo Researchers, Inc.: p. 17; © L. Birmingham/Custom Medical Stock Photo: p. 20; © Reuters/CORBIS: p. 24; © Clouds Hill Imaging Ltd./CORBIS: p. 25; © Mark Adams/SuperStock: p. 28; © St. Bartholomew's Hospital, London/Photo Researchers, Inc.: p. 32; © AP/Wide World Photos: pp. 39, 96; © Royalty-Free/CORBIS: pp. 41, 63, 64; © Mark Richards/CORBIS: p. 44; © Justin Sullivan/Getty Images: p. 45; © Lester Lefkowitz/CORBIS: pp. 55, 57; © Mediscan/Visuals Unlimited: p. 58; © Mauro Fermariello/Photo Researchers, Inc.: p. 59; © James Cavallini/Photo Researchers, Inc.: p. 60; © George Loun/Visuals Unlimited: p. 67; © Robert Llewellyn/SuperStock: p. 68; © Science VU/Visuals Unlimited: p. 69; © Owen Franken/CORBIS: p. 72; © Vo Trung Dung/CORBIS SYGMA: p. 73; © Layne Kennedy/CORBIS: p. 74; © Gabe Palmer/CORBIS: p. 81; © age fotostock/SuperStock: p. 85; © Jeffrey Greenberg/Photo Researchers, Inc.: p. 89 © Jon Feingersh/CORBIS: p. 90; © Hank Morgan/Photo Researchers, Inc.: p. 93

Copyright © 2006 by Alvin and Virginia Silverstein and Laura Silverstein Nunn

Twenty-First Century Books
A division of Lerner Publishing Group
241 First Avenue North
Minneapolis, Minnesota 55401 U.S.A.

Website address: www.lernerbooks.com

Library of Congress Cataloging-in-Publication Data

Silverstein, Alvin.
    Heart disease / by Alvin Silverstein, Virginia Silverstein & Laura Silverstein Nunn.
        p.   cm.—(Twenty-first century medical library)
    Includes bibliographical references and index.
    ISBN-13: 978-0-7613-3420-0 (lib. bdg. : alk. paper)
    ISBN-10: 0-7613-3420-3 (lib. bdg. : alk. paper)
        1. Heart—Diseases—Juvenile literature. I. Silverstein, Virginia B.
    II. Nunn, Laura Silverstein. III. Title. IV. Series.
    RC673.S556 2006
    616.1'2—dc22   2005004161

Manufactured in the United States of America
1 2 3 4 5 6 – BP – 11 10 09 08 07 06

CONTENTS

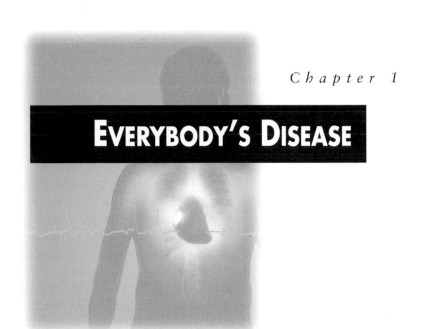

Chapter 1

EVERYBODY'S DISEASE

JESSICA'S STORY

Heart disease is something that old people get, right? That's what most people think. But New Jersey teenager Jessica Melore found out that it can happen to anyone. As a sixteen-year-old high school student, Jessica was bright, popular, outgoing, and athletic. She was an avid tennis player and seemed to be generally healthy. Then one day, celebrating her aunt's birthday at a restaurant, Jessica suddenly became dizzy. Her arms felt heavy, and pain seemed to be pressing out from her chest up to her neck. Her parents called 9-1-1, and an ambulance rushed Jessica to a hospital. The doctors at the emergency room said she was having a heart attack!

Tests showed that a large blood clot was blocking a major artery leading to Jessica's heart. Emergency surgery to clear out the clot didn't help; neither did another operation to bypass the block by attaching other arteries to the heart muscle. Jessica's heart was failing, and her lungs were filling up with fluid. The doctors told her parents that Jessica probably would not survive, and they called a priest to give her last rites. Though Jessica did make it through the crisis, her heart was badly damaged. A left ventricular assist device, or LVAD (a mechanical pump), helped to keep her alive through the long wait for a heart transplant.

It took more than nine months for a matching donor heart to become available. A few days before she was to graduate from high school, Jessica got a new heart—and a new lease on life. Four years later, Jessica was one of the American Heart Association volunteers who gathered in Washington in May 2003 to ask their senators to support more funding for research on heart disease and stroke. She spoke eloquently about her own experiences as a young heart-transplant survivor. Then she returned home for another important event—her graduation from Princeton University, after a "fairly typical, active and rewarding four years" in college.

AMERICA'S #1 KILLER

Heart disease is currently the number one killer in developed countries, and a rapidly growing health problem in Third World nations as well. In the United States, diseases of the heart and blood vessels account for close to two-thirds of the deaths each year—more than 700,000 deaths in 2000. Actually, the vast majority of heart disease patients *are* middle-aged or elderly. But many teenagers, children, and even newborn infants are affected as well.

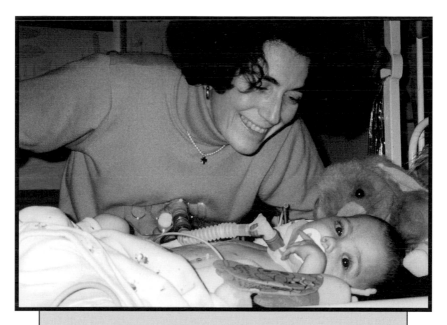

Young people are affected by heart disease, too. This baby was in dire need of a heart transplant when doctors said she only had hours to live. A donor was found and the transplant operation was successful.

Heart disease is not a single condition. It actually refers to any condition in which the heart and blood vessels are damaged in some way and are unable to function normally, which may lead to serious health problems and even death. For years, it was widely believed that heart disease was an illness that developed in adulthood. Recently, however, researchers have found that it may actually begin as early as the teen years. Many teenagers don't think twice about loading up on fatty foods such as double cheeseburgers and french fries or spending their afternoons playing video games instead of playing sports with their friends. If these unhealthy habits continue, they may take their toll on the body. Over time, fatty deposits start to clog up the artery walls, which could eventually lead to heart disease. Most cases of heart disease develop over a period of many years, and people may not notice symptoms until they are in their fifties or sixties.

Some kinds of heart disease are heart defects that are present at birth. If left untreated, they can greatly limit a child's activities and lead to an early death. Undetected heart defects may also cause a young person's heart to fail suddenly under the extra stress of competitive sports or other strenuous activities. In Jessica's case, she was very athletic and seemed to be in great physical condition, but nothing could have prevented a sudden heart attack that resulted from an unsuspected defect—a tiny hole in her heart. Some cases of heart disease are due to cardiomyopathy (an enlargement and weakening of the heart muscle, usually due to an infection or genetic change) that has gone undetected until too late. Heart problems often occur as a result of diabetes, which is becoming much more common today, especially among young people.

Odds are that you know somebody who has heart problems, or maybe you've heard about heart-attack victims on the radio or on TV. Anyone can be affected by heart disease, either directly or indirectly. Illness or death of parents, grandparents, and other loved ones can have tremendous effects on the entire family.

PROMISING PROGRESS

Fortunately, a lot of progress has been made in detecting, treating, and preventing cardiovascular disease, which refers to conditions involving the heart ("cardio") and blood vessels ("vascular"). A vast assortment of drugs can be used to control high blood pressure and high levels of "bad cholesterol," which can lead to heart and circulatory problems. Transplants and artificial blood vessels, heart valves, assist pumps, and even a full artificial heart provide

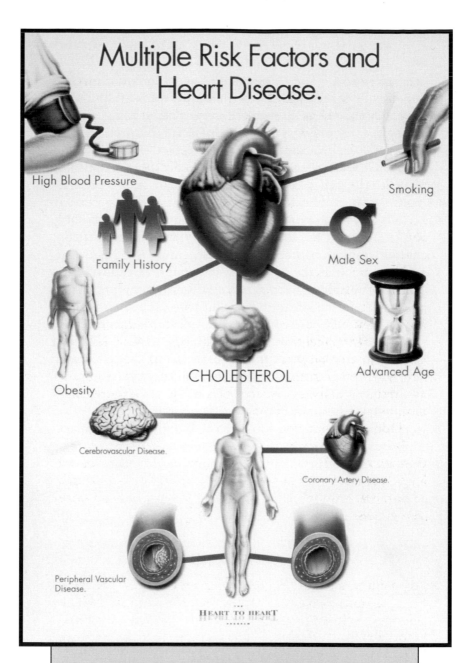

This poster from the National Institutes of Health shows that there are many causes of heart disease.

second chances for people with severe heart damage. Extensive research has shown that a person's lifestyle can have serious effects on the cardiovascular system. Obesity (being greatly overweight), which affects millions of children in the United States, increases a person's risk of developing cardiovascular problems. Medical experts agree that a well-balanced diet and exercise can help to keep the heart strong and healthy.

Meanwhile, researchers are gaining new insights into the causes of heart disease. Recently they have realized that inflammation of the blood vessels apparently plays an important role in the series of events that can lead to heart failure or a sudden heart attack. Anti-inflammatory treatments—the same kinds of drugs doctors use for asthma or arthritis—could be used to prevent and treat heart disease.

Thanks to new drugs and technology, as well as better education and healthier lifestyles, the heart disease death rate has been going down for a number of years.

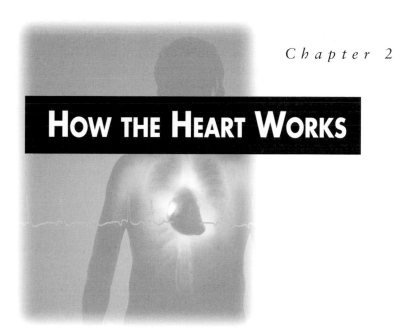

Chapter 2

HOW THE HEART WORKS

Do you know where your heart is? Many people think that it is on the left side of their chest. That's because when we pledge allegiance to the flag, we are taught to place our right hand over our heart—on the left side of the chest. Actually, however, the heart is in the middle of the chest. It fits nicely between the two lungs. But the heart is tipped, so that there is a little more of it on the left side than on the right. The pointed tip at the bottom of the heart touches the front wall of the chest. Every time the heart beats, it goes *thump* against the chest wall. You can feel your heartbeat when you put your hand over your chest, and you can hear a friend's heartbeat if you put your ear to his or her chest.

The heart has a very important job—it sends blood throughout the body to carry oxygen and important nutrients to all the body's cells. The blood can reach every part of your body through a system of tubes called blood vessels. The blood circulates around the body over and over again, which is why the heart and blood vessels are called the circulatory system. When something goes wrong in any part of the circulatory system, the heart is affected, too. If the blood vessels get clogged with fat deposits, for example, the tubes through which the blood flows become narrowed. Then the heart must work harder to keep the blood flowing through them. This puts a strain on the heart and makes it "wear out" faster.

Before we can understand how heart disease develops, we need to learn more about how the heart and blood vessels work and what they need to stay healthy.

HOW THE BLOOD CIRCULATES

If the blood vessels in our circulatory system were stretched out end to end, they would reach over 62,000 miles (nearly 100,000 km). That's enough to go around the earth more than twice! Inside the body, the blood vessels are linked into a complicated system. It takes less than a minute for the blood to circulate all around the body, and this happens about a thousand times a day. The blood continually gives the body cells the oxygen and nutrients they need. It also gets rid of the cells' waste products, such as carbon dioxide.

The heart is a muscle. And like any muscle in your body, the heart contracts (tightens). When this happens, it acts as a pump, sending blood rushing out through the blood vessels. We really have two circulatory systems. The pulmonary circulation is a short loop from the heart to the lungs and back again. The systemic circulation provides blood to all parts of the body. Both systems start and end at the heart, but there is no mixing between them.

Blood flows away from the heart in thick, muscular blood vessels called arteries. The biggest one, called the *aorta*, is an inch wide. These arteries soon branch out into

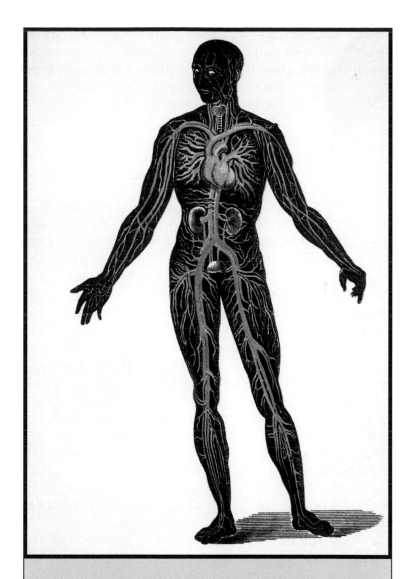

The heart is part of a very complicated system that circulates blood throughout the entire body. The system of arteries and veins that bring the blood to and from the heart is shown here.

smaller and smaller blood vessels. The tiniest blood vessels are called *capillaries*. Capillaries are so small they can be seen only with a microscope. Nearly every living cell in the body has a capillary near it. Oxygen and other nutrients pass through the capillary walls into the cells. Waste products pass from the cells into the capillaries. These waste products are brought back to the heart as the capillaries join to form tiny veins. As these veins get closer to the heart, they become larger, and eventually they empty into the heart. So the blood vessels of the body carry blood in a circle: moving away from the heart in arteries, traveling to various parts of the body in capillaries, and going back to the heart in veins.

There are blood vessels leading to all major organs and areas in the body. For each major artery carrying blood to an area, there is usually a vein draining blood away from it. Blood vessels are like the plumbing in a house. The body's pipes need to be kept free of clogs so that the blood can flow freely to all the parts of the body.

WHAT COLOR IS YOUR BLOOD?

If you cut your finger, the blood that spills out is red. Actually, it is the oxygen in the air that makes blood look red. In systemic circulation, arteries carry bright red, oxygen-rich blood, but veins carry purplish, oxygen-poor blood. The opposite occurs in pulmonary circulation.

THE HEART PUMP

The heart is like two pumps in one. A wall of muscle, called a *septum*, divides the heart into a left half and a right half—each side pumping at the same time. Another septum separates the rounded top part of the heart from the cone-shaped bottom part. So there are actually four chambers (areas) inside the heart. Each top chamber is called an *atrium* (atria *pl.*). The bottom chambers are called *ventricles*. Blood can flow from the atria down into

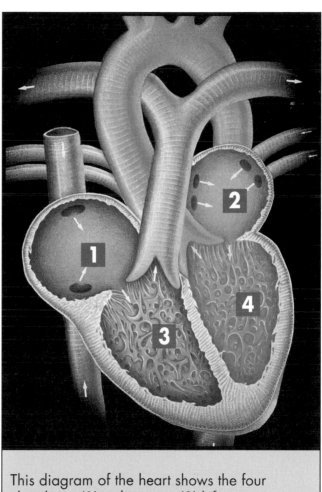

This diagram of the heart shows the four chambers: (1) right atrium (2) left atrium (3) right ventricle (4) left ventricle.

WHAT IS A HEARTBEAT?

A heartbeat is actually the sound your heart makes when it contracts. When the heart beats, you will hear two sounds—a long *lub* sound, quickly followed by a *dub* sound. These sounds are made when little trapdoors inside the heart snap shut to keep the blood from flowing backward. A newborn baby's heart beats about 120 times each minute. As we grow older, our heartbeat slows down. A child's heartbeat rate may be from 80 to 100 times a minute. An adult's heart beats an average of 70 times a minute.

You can find out your heart rate by taking your pulse. Contractions in the arteries help to move the blood along, creating a rhythmic throbbing on the surface of the skin. You can take your pulse by gently pressing two fingers against the inside of your other wrist until you feel a regular throbbing. (Don't use your thumb, which has a strong pulse of its own that could confuse you.) You can also check your pulse by putting two fingers on either side of your neck, just under the jawbone.

the ventricles, because there are openings in the walls that separate them. But blood cannot flow back and forth between the left and right halves of the heart. The septum that separates them is solid.

The right side of the heart is the receiver. It receives the "used up" blood from the body, which contains the cells' waste products (carbon dioxide, etc.). This blood is then pumped down to the lungs, where it picks up new, oxygen-rich blood and gets rid of the carbon dioxide and other waste products. (Carbon dioxide is removed from the blood when we breathe out.) At the same time, the left side of the heart receives the fresh, oxygen-rich blood from the lungs and then pumps it throughout the body. The left side of the heart has to work harder than the right because it has to pump blood to the farthest parts of the body. Every day, your heart pumps almost 2,000 gallons (7,500 L) of blood around your body.

When the heart contracts, the space inside it decreases. There is less room for blood, which goes gushing out through openings into arteries. The pumping action of the heart increases the pressure on the blood. The muscular walls in the arteries contract, too, maintaining the high pressure on the blood that keeps it flowing along. The blood pressure in the arteries can be measured by placing an inflatable cuff around the arm and listening to the sounds of the blood flowing through a large artery that lies close to the surface of the elbow.

The blood always flows in one direction—it never backtracks. That's because there are special "trapdoors," called valves, that separate the atria and the ventricles. The heart valves are actually movable flaps of tissue that keep blood from flowing backward. So, there is always one-way traffic in the heart.

The heart has four main valves. The *mitral valve* controls the blood flow from the left atrium to the left ventricle. The *tricuspid valve* controls the blood flow from the right atrium to the right ventricle. The *aortic valve*, which is very strong, controls blood flow from the left ventricle into the aorta (the large artery that sends blood throughout the body). The *pulmonary valve* controls the blood flow from the right ventricle to the pulmonary artery, which leads to the lungs. Each heart valve snaps shut after letting just the right amount of blood flow from one place to the next.

The heart keeps pumping over and over, in a regular rhythm. But the heart can't contract on its own. Electric

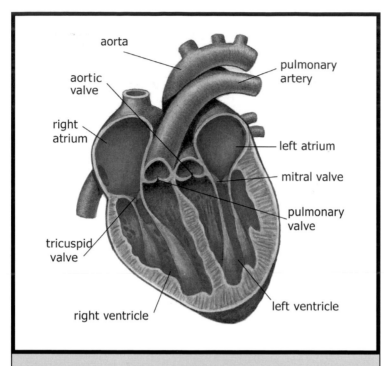

This side view of the heart shows all the valves and chambers.

signals keep it regular and set the rate of the rhythm. This is the body's own natural electricity, sent from specialized tissue in the heart muscle called the pacemaker. The amount of electricity is very tiny—not enough for you to even notice. A number of things can affect the rhythm of the heart. For example, when you are frightened or upset, your body sends out chemical messengers called *hormones* that make your heart beat faster. Sometimes being "scared to death" can cause palpitations—an uncomfortable thumping feeling in the chest, created by a racing heartbeat.

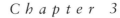

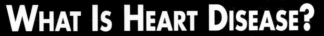

Chapter 3

WHAT IS HEART DISEASE?

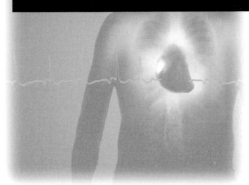

DOUG'S STORY

Doug had been an active person his whole life. Not even retirement could keep this sixty-six-year-old handyman from staying busy, building cabinets and sheds, repairing leaky faucets, and rewiring lights. Looking at him now, no one would realize that Doug had almost died of a heart attack several years earlier.

Doug's wife, Joan, always worried about her husband's need to "work, work, work." After all, both of his parents died from heart attacks—his mom at fifty-two and his dad at seventy-one. That meant that Doug had an increased risk for heart disease. But Doug did not want to slow down. Working with his hands made him feel young and alive. Then everything changed when Doug had his first heart attack, at age fifty-six. Fortunately, it was a mild one, and medicine and rest helped to nurse him back to health. But three years later, Doug had another heart attack. For a while it seemed like he was recovering from this one, too. Then things took a turn for the worse.

One morning, Doug woke with his lungs filled with fluid. He could hardly breathe, and he had trouble walking. Joan brought him to the emergency room. After taking X-rays, the doctors told Doug that he had an enlarged heart. Over the next several months, Doug went back and forth to the hospital for evaluations. But his condition only got worse. Doug was no longer the lively, energetic guy Joan once knew. Now her husband looked frail, and he could barely walk across the room, dress himself, or even eat. Doug's heart was badly damaged, and his only hope was a heart transplant. Without it, he would not survive. Doug was put on the heart-transplant list, but he was told it could be a long while before they could find a suitable donor. Fortunately, Doug's blood type was A-positive, which is common; this could help speed up the search for a match.

Amazingly, Doug had to wait only twenty days. Many patients have to wait for more than a year. In fact, a couple of Doug's friends had died while waiting for a heart. Doug knew how lucky he was. The new heart, which came from a nineteen-year-old on a respirator, gave Doug another chance at life. Now, with a new, healthy heart, Doug is once again back to his active self.

WHO GETS HEART DISEASE?

Doug's story seems to fit the picture that many people have about heart disease. We tend to think of heart disease as a condition that strikes mainly men over the age of fifty.

It is true that older men make up the majority of heart disease cases. However, more and more women are getting heart attacks than ever before. In fact, heart disease is the number one killer among women as well as men. A man's risk for heart disease increases after age forty-five. A woman's risk increases somewhat later, after about fifty-five years of age.

Heart disease may also strike children, teenagers, and young adults, although it is rare at these ages. Strangely, an increasing number of young people are having heart attacks. Undetected heart defects are often to blame. Young athletes with such defects are especially vulnerable to heart attacks because of the added stress on their bodies. There have been a number of highly publicized cases of heart disease affecting young athletes, including high school students such as Jessica, and even famous people such as Sergei Grinkov (Olympic ice skater), Darryl Kile (St. Louis Cardinals pitcher), and Reggie Lewis (Boston Celtics basketball player).

HOW HEART DISEASE DEVELOPS

In a young child, the insides of the arteries are smooth and slippery. Blood flows through them easily. Over time, little lumps of fatty material may stick to places inside the arteries. These little fatty patches are called plaques. As the years go by, the fatty plaques may grow bigger. Calcium salts may be added to them. Then they become hard, like bits of rock. This "hardening of the arteries" is known as *atherosclerosis*, a process that is responsible for most heart-disease cases. Atherosclerosis does not usually start to cause heart problems until middle or old age. But the plaques begin to build up much earlier, even in the teen years.

When atherosclerosis occurs, the arteries cannot work as well as they should. They are clogged up with plaques, so the opening for the blood to flow through gets narrower and narrower. Their walls become stiff and hard, so they

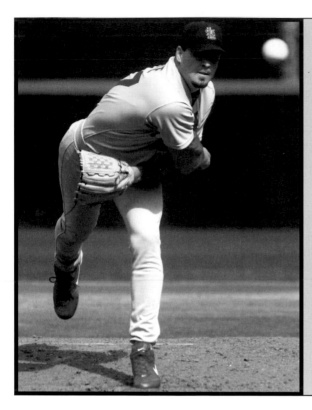

Heart disease can be fatal to athletes because of the added stress on their bodies. St. Louis Cardinals pitcher Darryl Kile died in 2002 at the age of 33 due to a narrowing of the arteries that supply the heart muscle. This is called coronary atherosclerosis.

cannot pump the blood along as well as they used to. When the arteries are hard and clogged, the heart has to work harder to pump blood through them. The heart may grow larger, trying to pump enough blood through the stiff arteries. It may become so large that it cannot get back to its normal size, the way it should.

When the coronary arteries—which carry oxygen-rich blood to the heart—get clogged with plaques, not enough blood can flow to the heart muscle. The heart cells do not get all the oxygen they need. Then the person may experience angina—a sharp pain or intense pressure in the chest. (The full medical name is *angina pectoris*.) Angina is a "call for help" from the starved heart cells. Hard work,

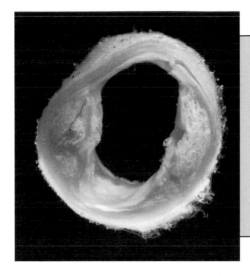

This is a section of an aorta that has atherosclerosis. The plaque is on the left and right of the aortic cavity.

exercise, or excitement may make the pain worse. That's because the heart is trying to work harder and needs even more oxygen than usual. Angina usually goes away when exercise or activity stops. However, if the condition is not treated, the pain may get worse, and it may even occur when the person is resting.

As the arteries get narrower and harder, the space inside them where blood flows through gets smaller and smaller. Eventually an artery may close up completely. Or, even more likely, a small blood clot may plug it up.

If you cut yourself, a blood clot can save your life. Your blood contains platelets, blood-clotting cells that stick to the edges of a damaged blood vessel. The platelets start to pile up until they form a plug that fills the hole. That stops the bleeding. Without platelets, we could bleed to death from a very small cut.

Blood clots are not supposed to happen *inside* a blood vessel. But plaques are rough. Sometimes they tear the delicate blood platelets inside a blood vessel, and then a clot may form inside. This kind of blood clot, called a *thrombus*, is dangerous.

There are chemicals in the blood that break up blood clots. Usually these chemicals take care of stray clots before they can do any harm. But if plaques have made the arteries very narrow, a clot may stick in a narrow spot and plug it up. Then no blood can flow past the plug.

What happens then? That depends on where the plug formed. Sometimes nothing happens. Many parts of the body get blood from several different arteries. If one gets plugged up, the cells will still get the oxygen and food materials they need from the other arteries. But some parts of the body have only one blood supply. If that artery is blocked, the cells will be starved. If the plug is not cleared away quickly, cells will start to die. This is called *infarction*. A myocardial infarction is the medical term for heart attack. ("Myocardial" comes from "myocardium," which is the medical name of the heart muscle.)

If a plug forms in one of the coronary arteries that supply the heart, part of the heart muscle will die. That is what happens in a heart attack. If only a small part of the heart muscle is hurt, the heart can keep on working. But it may not work as well as it used to. That's why people who have a heart attack have a greater risk of having a second one. When this happens, there may not be enough healthy heart muscle left to keep on beating.

STROKE: A BRAIN ATTACK

A heart attack happens when the heart's blood supply is cut off by a blood clot blocking an artery leading to the heart. If the blood supply to part of the brain is cut off, a person may have a "brain attack," better known as a stroke. Without the important oxygen and nutrients they need, brain cells will starve and die. This may happen when an artery leading to the brain is blocked by atherosclerosis, a blood clot, or an air bubble. It can also occur if a blood vessel in the brain ruptures and bleeds into the brain tissue. (A weak spot in a blood vessel, which may bulge out like a balloon and finally burst, is called an *aneurysm*.)

The brain is the control center for all of our thoughts, speech, and movements. When particular brain cells are damaged, this can affect a person's ability to speak or to move an arm or even one whole side of the body. If the blocked artery is treated quickly and the damage is not significant, the effects, such as slurred speech or weakness in the hands or feet, will be temporary. When brain cells die, they cannot grow back, but the remaining ones do have an amazing ability to form new connections and eventually return the body to normal functioning. Often a patient must "relearn" how to walk, speak, or even move a finger. However, if too many brain cells die, they will not be able to compensate for the loss, and permanent paralysis may result on one or both sides of the body. If the stroke affects the part of the brain that controls important body functions such as breathing, the person may die.

Strokes are most common among the elderly, but like heart attacks, they can strike at any age. Stroke is the third leading cause of death in the United States, and it is the number one cause of disability in adults.

CORONARY ARTERY DISEASE

Coronary artery disease (CAD) is the most common type of heart disease. It is usually caused by atherosclerosis, and it develops when one or more of the coronary arteries are narrowed or completely blocked by a gradual buildup of fatty plaques. The coronary arteries provide the heart with a constant supply of oxygen so it can keep pumping blood effectively. But when atherosclerosis affects one of these arteries, blood flow to the heart may be greatly reduced or even stopped. Then the heart doesn't get the important oxygen and nutrients it needs, and the person may develop angina, breathing problems, or other symptoms.

HEART ATTACKS

Many people think that heart disease and a heart attack are the same thing. Heart disease includes a number of different conditions that affect the heart and blood vessels. A heart attack is actually the *result* of certain kinds of heart disease, such as CAD. A heart attack happens when a

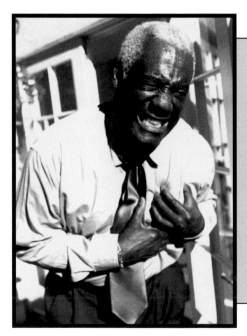

Many people describe the pain of a heart attack as intense, crushing pressure, as though an elephant were sitting on their chest. Sometimes the pain may shoot from the chest down one arm.

WHAT CAN TRIGGER A HEART ATTACK?

People can live for years not knowing their arteries are getting clogged with fat deposits. Yet a heart attack is sudden. What is the "last straw" that triggers it? Typically, it is a sudden exertion by someone who is not usually very physically active—for example, a person who works sitting at an office desk all week and then plays a few fast sets of tennis on the weekend. Carrying heavy packages up stairs can also bring on a heart attack. Shoveling snow can be particularly dangerous because the exertion is combined with extreme cold, which may trigger spasms (sudden, uncontrolled contractions) in the coronary arteries that cut off the blood flow to the heart muscle.

Other possible heart-attack triggers include:

- Extreme emotional stress

- Tobacco smoke

- Strenuous exercise

- Use of stimulant drugs such as cocaine or amphetamines

coronary artery is suddenly blocked, usually by a blood clot. This condition is called a *coronary thrombosis*, or coronary for short. Without oxygen-rich blood, starved heart cells start to die. Gradually, fibers of the damaged part stop contracting and die. A heart attack, or *myocardial infarction*—damage to or death of a portion of the heart muscle—has occurred.

In a heart attack, damage to the heart is permanent, but how serious it is depends on one main thing—time.

Sometimes the difference between life and death can be a matter of minutes. Some of the deadliest cases of heart attacks happen when the lack of oxygen affects the heart's own electrical system. When blood is not being pumped around the body, the heart starts to quiver rapidly. This is called *ventricular fibrillation*. Unless the normal rhythm of heart contractions is restored within a few minutes, cardiac arrest occurs—the heart stops. There is no heartbeat, no pulse, and no blood pressure. Unless medical help is provided immediately, sudden death could follow. Without the continuing supply of oxygen and nutrients that the blood carries throughout the body, various organs soon start to fail. The brain is one of the heaviest users of oxygen and sugar (the main nutrient used by the cells to generate energy). Brain cells will die in just four minutes unless the heart starts pumping again. If too many brain cells die, the heart-attack victim will die. Failure of the kidneys and other key organs can also contribute to disability or death after a heart attack.

CONGESTIVE HEART FAILURE

When the heart is not working properly, it isn't pumping blood around the body the way it's supposed to. Congestive heart failure occurs when the heart falls behind in its work, and it has trouble pumping enough blood to meet the body's needs. Blood is still being returned from various parts of the body, but less blood leaves the heart with each heartbeat. So the blood trying to enter the heart gets backed up. As a result, the pressure in the heart and blood vessels increases, which causes fluid from the blood to seep into surrounding tissues. This buildup of extra fluid in the tissues is called *congestion* (hence the name "congestive heart failure"). A person's legs, ankles, face, and hands may get puffy and swollen. Fluid may get into the lungs, making it harder to breathe. The kidneys may be affected as well. Normally, the job of the kidneys is to clean waste products and poisons out of the blood. But if the heart does not send enough blood through the kidneys, they cannot clean the blood. Some poisons stay in the blood and are carried to the cells. This can make the person really sick. Congestive heart failure can develop when the heart muscle has been damaged by a heart attack, infection, atherosclerosis, or high blood pressure.

HEART FAILURE OR HEART ATTACK?

People often think that heart failure and heart attack mean the same thing. Actually, a heart attack is a sudden event that results when the blood supply to the heart muscle is cut off. If a large part of the muscle is damaged, the heart stops beating. Without immediate help, the person may die. Heart *failure* doesn't mean that the heart stops, as many people think. It just means that the heart is not working properly. Congestive heart failure may develop slowly and gradually, but it can be just as dangerous as a heart attack. Without enough blood to nourish them, important body organs may be damaged and fail, too. If congestive heart failure is not treated, the person gradually becomes unable to do normal things like walking or carrying packages. Even breathing is a constant struggle. Eventually, the overburdened heart may give up, and the person dies.

HEART DEFECTS

Each year, about 35,000 babies in the United States are born with some heart problem. Most of these heart defects are mild. Conditions that are already present at birth are referred to as *congenital*. Congenital heart defects may be inherited, or they may be the result of something that happened while the baby was developing inside the mother. In rare cases, drugs taken by the mother or an infection such as German measles (rubella) may be responsible, but in most cases, doctors do not know what caused a congenital heart defect. The most common congenital heart problem is a hole in the septum, the wall that separates the two sides of the heart. Babies with this problem are often called blue babies because oxygen-rich blood mixes with oxygen-poor blood, giving their skin a bluish color. Doctors can repair this and other heart defects through surgery.

The hearts of children and adolescents may become damaged if a strep throat infection leads to rheumatic fever. Rheumatic fever can thicken and scar the heart valves, so blood does not flow properly through the heart and the

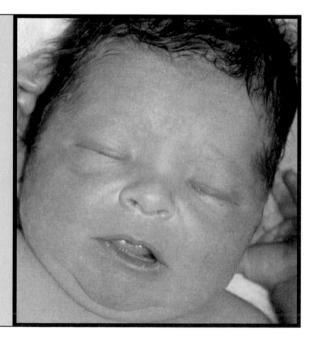

This baby is suffering from a congenital heart defect that results in deoxygenated blood being circulated throughout the body. The defect can be corrected immediately through surgery.

heart has to work harder. Rheumatic heart disease can be prevented by testing for strep whenever a child has a bad sore throat, and treating the infection with antibiotics.

Kawasaki disease is another infection that can lead to serious heart problems. This illness affects very young children, usually under five years old. Typical symptoms include a high fever; a rash; swollen hands, feet, and glands; and red, swollen lips, mouth, and throat. Most children who contract Kawasaki disease recover quickly with proper medical care. About 20 percent of them, however, develop complications that can damage blood vessels and weaken the heart.

Most people have heart murmurs at some point in their lives. A heart murmur is a hissing or swishing sound between the *lub, dub* sounds of a heartbeat. Usually, it is just the sound of blood rushing through the heart and is perfectly normal. But sometimes a heart murmur can be a sign of a serious problem, one that a person was born with or that was caused by an illness. For example, the heart may have a hole in it, and the heart murmur may be the sound of blood going in and out of the hole. Or it could be a sign of a leaky heart valve, or possibly a valve that does not open all the way.

CARDIOMYOPATHY

Cardiomyopathy is a serious heart condition in which the heart muscle is damaged and loses its ability to pump blood effectively. Damage to the heart muscle may be caused by a heart attack, as we have seen, but some viral infections can also attack the heart. Alcohol use can damage the heart muscle, as well. In some cases, doctors cannot find a specific cause, but many of these may be due to an inherited defect that is unsuspected until a sudden, extreme exertion puts extra stress on the heart. Such a genetic defect is usually the underlying cause when an apparently healthy young athlete suddenly collapses with a heart attack during a sports competition. About 50,000 Americans are diagnosed with cardiomyopathy each year. Many of them are much younger than the typical person with heart disease. It can affect young adults, teenagers, and even children.

Cardiomyopathy can take several different forms. The heart muscle may become weak, and the chambers inside the heart become enlarged and stretched out. This condition may be present for years without showing any symptoms. But gradually, as the heart weakens, it falls behind in its pumping work and congestive heart failure may develop. Enlargement of the heart may also be produced by a thickening of the heart muscle. This is not the normal enlargement that occurs in the heart of a highly trained athlete, making the heart's pumping more effective. Instead, some parts of the heart may enlarge more than others. When the septum between the two ventricles enlarges, it may partly block the flow of blood out of the left ventricle into the blood vessels that feed the body. Thickening can also distort the heart valves, causing them to leak and producing a heart murmur. In some cases of cardiomyopathy, the heart muscle becomes stiff and the heart cannot fill with blood effectively. Thus there is not enough blood to pump with each heartbeat.

Cardiomyopathy can also lead to *arrhythmia*, an unusual or irregular heartbeat. Sometimes an arrhythmia may be a sign of a problem with the heart's electrical system. Normally, the body's natural pacemaker sends out tiny bursts of electricity to signal the heart that it needs to pump blood. But if the pacemaker is not working properly, the heartbeat may become too slow (a condition called *bradycardia*). Or it may become irregular, skipping a beat from time to time. Then the body isn't getting the important oxygen and nutrients it needs, which could lead to symptoms such as exhaustion, dizziness, or lightheadedness.

SIGNS OF HEART TROUBLE

Heart disease usually takes years to develop, and people may not experience any symptoms until after fifty years of age. Generally, symptoms start to show up after the space inside the arteries has narrowed more than 50 percent. Sometimes a heart attack seems to come out of the blue, striking someone without any previous symptoms. But in most cases, there are usually obvious signs of trouble. Too often people tend to ignore these signs, thinking that they have indigestion, or that their aches and pains will go away. If these symptoms are caught early and treated, a heart attack can be avoided.

It is not always easy to identify signs of heart trouble. Symptoms may vary among individuals, and the signs may differ among the different types of heart disease. So how do people know whether the signs mean trouble? A number of key symptoms and signs are often associated with heart and blood-vessel disease. Anybody who has a combination of them should see a health-care provider. Here's what to look for:

- Chest pain (angina pectoris) or intense pressure in the chest

- Shortness of breath

- General fatigue (tiredness)

- Swelling (especially the legs and ankles)

- Loss of consciousness

- Dizziness or lightheadedness

- Palpitations

- Nausea or vomiting

- Sweating

- Limb pain or weakness

- Abnormal skin color

- Sores on skin

- Sudden change in vision, strength, coordination, speech, or sensation

As we mentioned earlier, heart disease is *not* just a men's disease. Women can also have heart attacks, but they generally develop symptoms about ten years later than men do. However, researchers have found that symptoms of heart disease are different in men and women. For example, men commonly complain about pressure in the left side of the chest, or pain shooting down one arm. Women may not have chest pain, but instead have a burning sensation in the upper abdomen or under the breastbone. Other possible symptoms may include fatigue, sleep disturbance, shortness of breath, sweating, nausea, vomiting, fainting, and lightheadedness. Often these signs are confused with indigestion or menopause or some other normal occurrence. Researchers say that these symptoms may show up as much as a month before the heart attack occurs. Now that doctors know that heart disease symptoms are sometimes different in women, they may be able to better prevent possible heart attacks.

Although heart disease strikes more men than women, women are more likely to die of the disease because of the difficulty in recognizing the symptoms. A recent study showed that only 10 percent of men having symptomatic heart attacks (heart attacks with previous symptoms) died within a year. However, as many as 45 percent of women having symptomatic heart attacks died within a year.

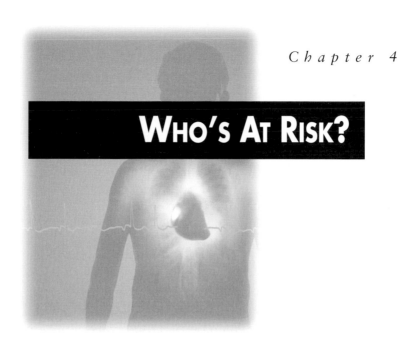

Chapter 4

WHO'S AT RISK?

SERGEI'S STORY

On November 20, 1995, people all over the world were shocked to learn that Olympic gold medalist Sergei Grinkov had died while training at an ice rink in Lake Placid, New York. Grinkov, who was only twenty-eight years old, died suddenly of a heart attack. His wife, Ekaterina Gordeeva, told the doctor at the hospital that he had never complained about any chest pains. Grinkov seemed to be in great shape and excellent health. The only known risk factor he had was that his father had died of a sudden heart attack at age fifty-two.

An autopsy revealed that Grinkov had severely clogged arteries. Doctors wondered how such a young, athletic man could develop arteries that looked like those of a seventy-year-old man with atherosclerosis. After reading about Grinkov's death in the New York Times, *Pascal J. Gold-schmidt of Johns Hopkins University thought he knew the answer to that question. Goldschmidt and his colleagues believed that a gene was to blame for Grinkov's condition. This gene, which produces a protein involved in blood clotting, comes in two forms, PIA1 and PIA2. The PIA2 form has been found to increase the risk of an early heart attack.*

The Hopkins research team managed to get a sample of Grinkov's blood and test it for this gene. The results showed that Grinkov did inherit the PIA2 form, most likely from his father. What probably happened, researchers theorized, was that a piece of fatty material clinging to the artery walls broke off and left a hole. The PIA2 gene in Grinkov's body became activated and started to form a small clot to plug up the hole. However, it overdid it, and formed a massive clot that plugged up the entire coronary artery, blocking the blood flow to the heart. Researchers believe that the same gene may also be responsible for speeding up atherosclerosis, which is usually a very slow process.

About 20 percent of the United States' population has the PIA2 gene. This doesn't mean that people with this gene will have a heart attack. It just increases the risk, or likelihood, that it will happen. In most cases, heart disease is caused by a combination of risk factors, not just one.

FAMILY HISTORY

Heart disease tends to run in families. People whose parents had a heart attack before the age of sixty have an increased risk for developing coronary artery disease. A recent study showed that people with at least one parent who had early heart disease tend to have thicker artery

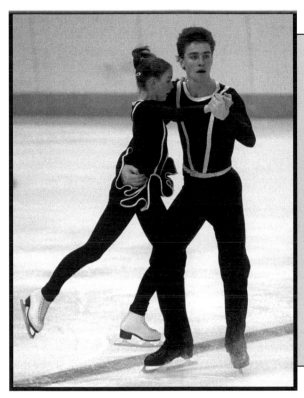

In Sergei Grinkov's case, the PIA gene, family history, and being an athlete (placing extreme stress on the body) became the deadly combination that led to his heart attack.

walls than the average person of the same age. This thickening is an indication that plaque is building up and atherosclerosis is developing. This study supports general observations that people with a family history of heart disease have a higher risk of having a heart attack than people who have no incidence of heart disease in their family.

Family is an important part of people's early environment. It has a strong influence on their lifestyle—how active they are, the kinds of foods they eat, and whether they smoke. But environment is only a small part of the family's role in determining heart-attack risk. Heredity may play an even greater role. The parents may pass on genes for high levels of cholesterol or other fatty materials (lipids) in the blood, as well as other risk factors such as high blood pressure, obesity, or diabetes.

A family history of heart disease may place a person at high risk for heart disease, but it is not an automatic death sentence. Lifestyle choices such as exercise and healthy eating habits can help to counteract hereditary influences.

HIGH CHOLESTEROL

We often hear people talk about cholesterol in connection with heart disease. What exactly is cholesterol? Cholesterol is a fatty substance that is found in foods from animal sources, such as meat, eggs, poultry, fish, and dairy products. It is also the main fatty material in the plaques that clog up arteries. Studies have shown that people with a lot of cholesterol in their blood are more likely to get heart attacks. But at the same time, our body needs cholesterol. For example, it is an important part of the brain and nerves. We get some of it in the foods we eat, but the body can make cholesterol, too. In fact, if you eat less cholesterol, your body may make more of it.

Scientists have found that the cholesterol in the blood becomes attached to certain types of fats: high-density lipoproteins (HDLs) and low-density lipoproteins (LDLs). HDL is the "good cholesterol." It helps to carry cholesterol out of the arteries to the liver and then out of the body. LDL is the "bad cholesterol." It deposits cholesterol in the inner linings of the arteries and contributes to plaque buildup. So when doctors measure cholesterol in the blood, they look at the HDL and LDL levels. The higher the HDL level, the better, and the lower the LDL, the better. The normal range for total blood cholesterol levels is 100 to 199 milligrams per deciliter of blood; at 200 and above, the risk of heart disease begins to rise. People with total cholesterol of 240 have twice the risk of a heart attack or stroke as those with a cholesterol level of 200.

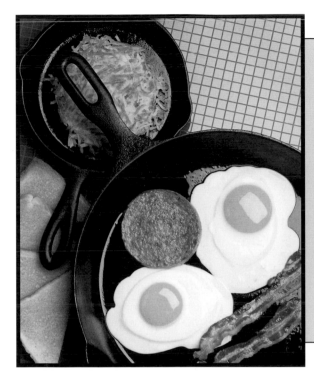

Eating too many foods that contain animal fats and cholesterol, such as meat and eggs, could increase the risk of developing heart disease.

The LDL level should be lower than 100, and the HDL level should be at least 40 or higher. A high total cholesterol level is not necessarily bad if the HDL level is high.

Most fats, both in foods and in the body, are in a chemical form called triglycerides. These fats are an important source of energy for the body. Excess calories from food are converted to triglycerides and stored in fat cells. They serve as energy reserves that the body can call on when it needs an energy boost. Triglycerides are transported through the blood mainly by very low-density lipoproteins (VLDLs). High levels of triglycerides in the blood are linked to atherosclerosis and heart disease. Doctors will check for triglycerides along with cholesterol levels. Normal levels of triglycerides are less than 200.

OBESITY AND PHYSICAL INACTIVITY

Eating too many calories from any type of food not only increases your cholesterol level, but it can also make you overweight, which is another important risk factor for heart disease. Obesity (being greatly overweight) is a serious problem in the United States, where people often have a diet that is high in fat and sugar. Obesity affects an estimated 15 percent of American kids between the ages of twelve and nineteen. And there is an 80 percent chance that those children will continue to be overweight into adulthood.

When a person gains weight, the body tends to make less HDL cholesterol and more LDL cholesterol and triglycerides. Obese people often develop diabetes and hypertension. Being overweight is also harmful because the heart has to work harder to pump blood through all that extra fatty tissue. The heart may eventually wear out and weaken, which could also lead to heart problems.

"NATURAL" ISN'T ALWAYS SAFE

Until recently, ephedra, an herbal supplement, was highly valued among athletes as a "natural" energy booster. It was used to help improve an athlete's performance in sports by enhancing strength and speed. It was also used for losing weight. But ephedra is not a harmless herb. It has been responsible for more than a hundred deaths.

Health officials have now labeled ephedra a drug, since this natural supplement can have serious effects on the body. It can speed up the heart rate, narrow blood vessels, and cause high blood pressure, which can lead to a heart attack. It can also cause severe dehydration that can be deadly, as well as health problems such as stroke, liver and kidney damage, and seizures. Some minor side effects may include nausea, diarrhea, and arrhythmia.

The Food and Drug Administration (FDA) had considered ephedra a food supplement, so it didn't have to be regulated. This meant that this herb could be sold anywhere—the supermarket, the mall, the Internet. A recent survey found that about a million kids between the ages of twelve and seventeen had taken this dangerous supplement.

In 2002, newspapers reported that a sixteen-year-old high school football player from Illinois died of a heart attack after taking ephedra, which he bought at a local gas station. His father said that he was taking the supplement to help make him a first-stringer on the football team. This story sparked a drive to ban ephedra and keep it out of the hands of young people. A number of states banned the sale of ephedra to children under eighteen years of age. Meanwhile, manufacturers of "energy boosting" supplements changed their formulas to make their products ephedra-free. In April 2004 the FDA banned most forms of ephedrine (the active drug in ephedra) in products sold without a prescription.

Exercise, along with a healthy diet with fewer calories, is a great way to eliminate excess weight and make the heart strong again. However, many kids are not getting as much exercise as their bodies need. More often, they spend

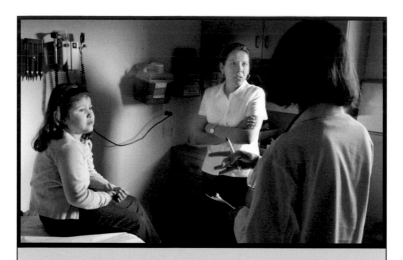

This four-year-old, who weighed 95 pounds (twice her ideal weight), became obese when she spent too much time watching television. Her doctor and mother have helped her learn to eat healthier foods and become more active.

their days watching TV, playing video games, or surfing the 'Net rather than getting a group of friends together and playing ball in the backyard. Physical inactivity and obesity often go hand in hand. When people are inactive, they are more likely to gain weight because they are not burning up as many calories as they take in. This could lead to obesity, and therefore it increases their risk for heart disease.

HIGH BLOOD PRESSURE

People who are overweight are also more likely to have high blood pressure, or *hypertension*. ("Hyper" means high, and "tension" refers to the pressure inside the arteries.) If the arteries become narrow, the heart has to pump more forcefully to push blood through them, which causes the blood pressure to go up. In other words, the heart has to work harder to pump the same amount of blood. Hypertension is a serious risk factor for heart disease. In fact, it is sometimes called the silent killer because there are usually no symptoms, and many people don't even know that they have it. Studies have found that too much salt in a person's diet can cause high blood pressure.

Blood pressure is expressed as two values: the *systolic pressure*, measured while the heart is contracting and pumping blood into the arteries (systole), and the *diastolic pressure*, measured when the heart is relaxed and its chambers are filling with blood (diastole). Blood pressure in the arteries is highest during systole, when blood from the heart is flooding into them. As the heart relaxes and stops forcing blood into the arteries, the pressure inside them drops—but not all the way to zero. During diastole, the

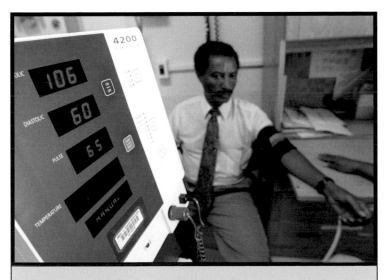

This machine shows that the man's blood pressure is in the normal range, with a reading of 106/60.

muscular artery walls still maintain some pressure on the blood flowing through them.

Blood pressure is measured in millimeters of mercury and is read in the form of a fraction; for example, 120/80, which is read as "120 over 80." The high number represents the systolic pressure, when the heart is contracting, and the low number is the diastolic pressure, when the heart is relaxed. The normal range of the systolic pressure in a healthy young adult at rest is 100 to 120. The diastolic pressure ranges from 60 to 80. A resting blood pressure above 140/90 is considered to be high blood pressure (hypertension).

DIABETES

Adults with diabetes are two to four times more likely to have a heart attack or a stroke than are people without diabetes. Diabetes is a condition in which not enough of the hormone insulin is produced, or it does not properly control the body's use and storage of glucose (sugar). As a result, abnormally high amounts of glucose stay in the blood. Having high blood sugar over a long period of time can damage the heart and blood vessels, which can speed up atherosclerosis and lead to increased blood levels of triglycerides, decreased levels of "good" HDL cholesterol, high blood pressure, and, eventually, a heart attack. At least 65 percent of people with type 2 diabetes (the most common kind, which typically occurs in adults) will suffer a heart attack or a stroke. Often, obesity plays a significant role in the development of this type of diabetes. Losing weight can greatly reduce blood-sugar levels, as well as decrease the risk of having a heart attack.

SMOKING

We've been told that smoking can cause cancer. But did you know that it is also bad for your heart? Heavy smok-

SECONDHAND SMOKE

When a cigarette smoker takes a puff and then
exhales, chemicals from the cigarette smoke are sent
into the air. Not only does the smoker breathe in
these poisons, but everyone around that person
does, too. So if you don't smoke but spend a lot of
time around someone who does, you are breathing
secondhand smoke. Inhaling somebody else's smoke
can give you the same kinds of health problems that
smokers develop.

ers are more than twice as likely to have heart attacks as
people who don't smoke.

Cigarettes contain thousands of different substances, a
number of which have harmful effects on the body. One of
the most important chemicals in cigarettes is nicotine. Nicotine is a powerful drug that acts on the heart and blood vessels. It speeds up the heart and makes it need more oxygen.
It also narrows the arteries, so that the heart has to pump
harder. Eventually, after many years of smoking, the heart
may become weakened by the extra strain. Smoking also
makes blood more likely to clot inside the blood vessels.

Cigarette smoke also contains carbon monoxide, the
same gas that is in car exhaust. This gas is picked up by
red blood cells that normally carry oxygen. The red blood
cells hold it so tightly that they can't let go, and they can
no longer carry oxygen. As a result, the body cells do not
get as much oxygen as they need. So smoking may cause
attacks of angina because the heart cells are starving.
These kinds of problems usually do not occur unless a person has smoked for many years, but smoking at a young
age can lead to serious heart conditions later in life.

STRESS

Stress may be another important risk factor in heart disease. When we are worried or upset, our bodies make a hormone called *adrenaline*. This is a chemical that speeds up the heart. It is adrenaline that makes us feel as if our heart is pounding out of our chest when we are frightened. Stress also makes the blood pressure go up, at least temporarily. Research suggests that people who react with anger to minor, everyday irritations may be at increased risk for a heart attack. More studies are needed on the role of stress in the development of heart disease.

INFLAMMATION

Until recently, the popular view of how heart disease develops was rather simple: high levels of cholesterol and triglycerides in the blood cause fatty deposits (plaque) to build up inside the arteries that supply the heart muscle, narrowing them and eventually plugging them up completely so that blood cannot get through. Research has now shown, however, that although narrowed coronary arteries can cause chest pains and other symptoms of heart disease, only about 15 percent of heart attacks actually happen this way—and about half of the people who have heart attacks had a normal blood cholesterol level! Evidence is building up to suggest that another body process plays a major role in heart attacks: inflammation.

You've probably had a cut or splinter that became infected. You may recall how the skin around it got red, hot, swollen, and very painful. These are the signs of inflammation, which is actually an important body defense against disease germs. Damage to body tissues prompts the release of chemical messengers that cause tiny blood vessels in the area to leak fluids into the tissues, causing them to swell. The chemical messengers also act as alarm signals that call in white blood cells, the body's roaming defenders and clean-up squad. Some white blood cells can identify "foreign" substances such as the chemicals on the outside of germs. Others attack invading germs and clear away bits of damaged cells. The fluid that leaks out of the blood into the tissues during inflammation makes it easier for the white blood cells to move around.

Usually inflammation is a brief reaction, which quiets down as the damage heals. But researchers are discovering that spots of long-term, chronic inflammation may develop inside the blood vessels. The problem tends to start when the body's defense systems detect plaques forming on the artery walls, and white blood cells go after them, trying to clear them away. The white cells burrow into the plaques, weakening them so that they may become inflamed, swell up, and suddenly tear apart and trigger the formation of blood clots. The plaques that cause trouble are not necessarily large ones but, rather, ones that are too small to block arteries on their own.

The new focus on the importance of inflammation is helping to explain some other parts of the heart-disease puzzle. Medical experts now realize, for example, that obesity does more than just make the heart work harder to pump blood through the extra flesh. Fat cells are not just storage depots for extra fuel. They are tiny factories that produce hormones and other chemical messengers that affect the whole body. Some of the chemicals that fat cells produce can cause inflammation, others promote the formation of blood clots, and still others cause the blood vessels to narrow and the blood pressure to rise.

Doctors have already begun to use tests for chemical indicators of inflammation to help predict heart-attack risk, and a number of companies are trying to develop tools and techniques for detecting the particular "hot spots" of inflammation that may lead to a heart attack or stroke.

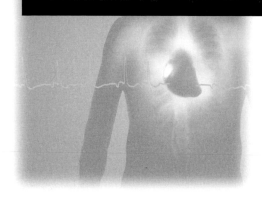

Chapter 5

DETECTING HEART PROBLEMS

JOHN'S STORY

John worked for a prestigious law firm as a high-powered attorney. For many years, he had worked hard to become well respected in his field. That meant long hours and a lot of take-out food. At age forty-eight, John had achieved his dream job, but he missed being with his family at night for dinner. John ordered takeout almost every night. He especially loved to eat Mexican food, but sometimes he got sharp pains in his chest shortly after eating it. When he chewed a couple of antacid tablets, the pain soon went away.

One day, John had pain in his chest again after eating Mexican food. But this time, the antacids did not seem to work. In fact, the pain was getting worse. About twenty minutes later, John started to sweat and he felt nauseous. Maybe it's food poisoning, he thought. He decided to lie down on the couch in his office for a few minutes, hoping he would feel better.

About an hour later, his friend and coworker, Mike, who also happened to be working late, came into John's office and saw him lying there, looking very pale and weak. John could hardly speak but was able to tell Mike that he was having trouble breathing, and felt like an elephant was sitting on his chest. Mike called 9-1-1 immediately. He explained the situation to the operator and waited for the ambulance. The symptoms seemed obvious—John was having a heart attack.

Mike called John's wife, Donna, to let her know what happened. Donna took their kids to stay at a neighbor's house, and then she rushed over to the hospital. When Donna got there, she saw John hooked up to an electrocardiograph (ECG) machine. This test can show if someone is actually having a heart attack, if the heart is damaged, and where the trouble is. The ECG confirmed that John was having a heart attack, but amazingly, his heart was not seriously damaged even though it had taken him a long time to get to the hospital after his first symptoms.

Like many people, John did not pay attention to the clues his body was giving him, and he refused to admit that he was building up risk factors for a heart attack. All his life he worked really hard, endured a great deal of stress, and took very little care of his body by spending a lot of time sitting behind a desk and not eating healthy meals. He also didn't like going to the doctor, so he rarely got checkups. If John had had an annual physical exam, the doctor might have detected existing health problems, and with proper treatment and some lifestyle changes, could have prevented his heart attack.

PHYSICAL EXAMINATION

We tend to think of a heart attack as sudden and intense, like those we see in the movies. A person clutches his or her chest and collapses to the floor. While a heart attack may appear sudden, however, it actually took years to get to this point. By now, you know that heart disease is generally a long process that may start to develop as early as the teen years. Therefore, medical experts recommend that even young people should have physical exams regularly. When it comes to heart disease, early detection is the key—before the arteries have had a chance to become so clogged with plaque that a heart attack could happen at any moment. People can have heart problems and not even know it. Only medical tests can show if they have serious risk factors, such as high blood pressure or high cholesterol levels.

Before starting the physical exam, a doctor needs to collect information about the patient, including any noticeable symptoms and family medical background. Since heart disease tends to run in families, it is especially important to find out if the patient's mother or father had heart disease.

A physical exam includes some simple tests for the heart and blood vessels. The doctor uses a stethoscope to listen to the patient's heartbeat. Heart murmurs or heart defects can be detected with this simple medical tool. The patient's pulse rate is also taken, usually by a nurse, which also helps to show if the heart is beating normally.

Blood pressure is measured using a device called a *sphygmomanometer*. An inflatable cuff is wrapped around the arm just above the elbow. When the cuff is inflated, it presses on the arteries in the arm and briefly closes them, cutting off the flow of blood to the lower arm. Then the air is slowly let out of the cuff while the doctor or nurse listens to the sounds coming from the artery with a stethoscope and watches a gauge connected to the cuff that measures the air pressure in the cuff. When the air pressure in the cuff falls just below the blood pressure in the artery, blood starts to flow through the artery again, and a pulse beat (a tapping sound) can be heard with the stethoscope. The reading on the gauge when the first beat is heard is the systolic pressure. As more air is let out of the cuff, the sound fades away completely; the pressure shown on the dial at that moment is the diastolic pressure.

Routine blood tests can also provide a lot of information. They can show a person's total cholesterol, as well as the individual levels of HDL, LDL, and triglycerides in the blood. It is best to fast before the blood test to get a more accurate reading. For people with risk factors for heart disease, the doctor will also order a newer test, called the CRP test. This test determines the level of a blood chemical called C-reactive protein (CRP). It is produced whenever inflammation is present in the body. A sprained ankle or a case of the flu will result in very high CRP values, but these will soon go down when the ankle heals or the body defeats the attacking flu viruses. Smaller, chronic increases in the CRP level that don't go away from one test to the next may be an indication of a longer-lasting health problem. A higher-than-normal CRP test by itself does not necessarily mean the person has heart disease. It may be due to another problem, such as arthritis, a condition involving painful swelling of the joints. The CRP test is just one part of the evidence that the doctor puts together to form a picture of the patient's health. If any of the test results seem suspicious, the person may be sent to a heart specialist, called a *cardiologist*.

Blood tests can also be used in emergency situations, to determine whether or not a person is having a heart attack. When the heart is damaged, certain enzymes and proteins are released into the bloodstream. Their amounts in the blood rise in the hours after a heart attack, reaching a peak after about twenty-four hours. These chemicals are "biomarkers" that can be detected in blood tests.

Increased levels of the biomarkers can confirm that a heart attack has occurred and indicate how badly the heart has been damaged. The test for a muscle protein called troponin is considered the most accurate.

HOW OFTEN DO YOU NEED A MEDICAL CHECKUP?

Regular medical checkups can help to detect developing problems before they get serious. Specialists at the Mayo Clinic recommend that people with no obvious health problems should have checkups at least:

- Every five years in their twenties
- Every three to four years in their thirties
- Every two to three years in their forties
- Every two years in their fifties
- Every year at age sixty or older

ELECTROCARDIOGRAPH (ECG)

One of the most important tools for checking on the health of the heart is the electrocardiograph, or ECG. By recording the electrical activity of the heart, an ECG can show the doctor if heart muscle is injured or overworked.

An ordinary ECG is given while the patient is lying down on a table, completely relaxed. Electrodes pasted on the chest and each arm and leg can pick up the heart's electricity. The electrical impulses are recorded in the form of waves that are shown on graph paper. The ECG can give a lot of important information about the heart and blood vessels, including the heart rate, heart rhythm, whether a heart attack has occurred, insufficient blood and oxygen supply to the heart, and heart structure abnormalities.

Sometimes heart problems don't show up until the heart is pumping hard. In a stress test, the patient may walk on a treadmill or pedal a stationary bike while the ECG records the heart's activity. Blood pressure is monitored as well. The doctor can look for abnormalities that take place over a whole day of normal activity by hooking up a tiny, lightweight ECG, called a Holter monitor, which the patient wears throughout the day. Electrodes are attached to the person's chest, hidden underneath the

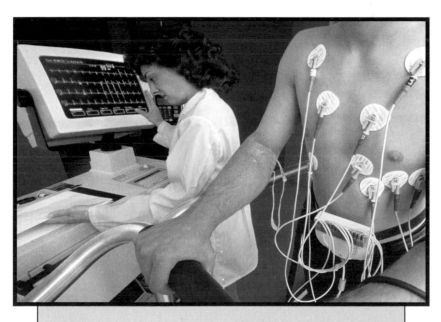

A stress test is being given while the doctor reads the ECG printout.

clothing, and a small tape recorder, which can be hooked to a belt or carried on a strap, makes a continuous recording of the ECG. The person also keeps a written log, noting the times for activities such as eating, walking, and playing sports. Later, the cardiologist can scan through the tape and look over an entire day's heart activity, comparing it to the written log.

CHEST X-RAYS

We often think of X-rays as a way to detect broken bones. X-rays can also give important information about vital organs, such as the heart and lungs. For example, a chest X-ray can show the size and shape of the heart. It can detect some congenital defects. It can also show whether the heart chambers are enlarged. (A failing heart may get larger as it struggles to pump enough blood.)

X-rays can also detect calcium deposits. Calcium is the main substance in bones. X-rays can't pass through calcium, which is why bones show up on film. Sometimes calcium deposits can be found in damaged heart muscle, diseased valves, or coronary arteries with atherosclerosis. Like bones, these calcium deposits can be seen on X-ray film.

To get a clearer picture of the heart, a cardiac catheter may be placed in a vein in the patient's arm. The long, thin, flexible tube (catheter) is slowly pushed along the bloodstream until it reaches the heart. The doctor can measure the blood pressure in the heart chambers and can find out whether the blood in the chambers has a normal amount of oxygen. By injecting a dye through the catheter, the doctor can take X-rays called *angiograms* that show how the dye moves through the blood vessels and heart chambers. An angiogram can give a clear picture of heart damage, valve leaks, and other problems, as well as reveal narrowing arteries.

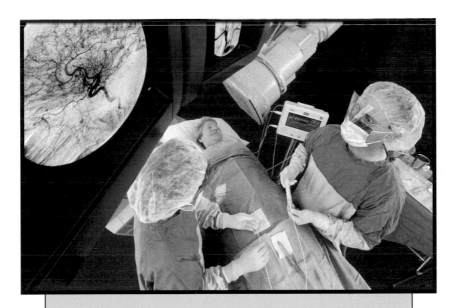

An angiogram is usually given after preliminary tests such as chest X-rays, an ECG, and blood tests detect heart problems. It may be used as a kind of road map for doctors to follow in case surgery is needed.

NUCLEAR SCANNING

While X-rays help to give an inside look at the structure of a person's heart, nuclear scanning is a diagnostic technique that can help doctors see how blood is pumped through the heart. In an X-ray, radiation passes through a person's body to produce an image. During a nuclear scan, tiny amounts of radioactive elements, called *radioisotopes*, are injected into the bloodstream. These "tracers" give off radiation (energy), which is picked up by a special camera that takes "photographs" as the radioisotopes make their journey through the heart. The images are then displayed on a computer. This allows the doctors to see whether blood is being pumped effectively through the heart. Some radioisotopes travel through the heart chambers, while others go directly to the heart muscle, where blood flow may be reduced due to coronary artery disease. Although injecting a radioactive substance into the body sounds dangerous, very tiny amounts are used in nuclear scans. Doctors consider this a safe and effective diagnostic tool.

SPECIALIZED IMAGING TESTS

The computerized axial tomography (CT or CAT) scan uses tiny streams of X-rays sent through the body at various angles to produce revealing pictures that are far clearer and more detailed than an ordinary X-ray image. The CT scan gives a detailed "slice," or cross-section view, of the body, including the heart, pericardium, lungs, and blood vessels. (The pericardium is a fluid-filled sac enclosing the heart.)

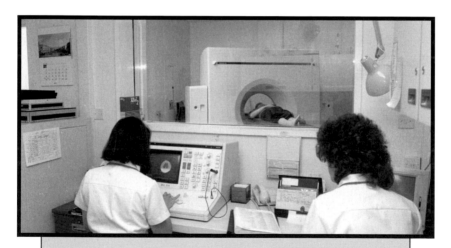

A patient undergoes a CT scan while the radiographers sit outside the scan room to protect themselves from the potentially harmful radiation.

During a CT scan, the machine rotates as it scans the person lying on the table. Since the heart is constantly in motion, the pictures may appear blurry. But a technique called the electron beam CT, often called the ultrafast CT, uses special instruments that can produce clear images. Now widely used, these fast CT scans can detect calcium deposits that may lead to CAD.

A magnetic resonance imaging (MRI) scan uses a strong magnetic field and radio waves that pass through the body to produce clear images of almost any organ in the body. It is more sophisticated than a CT scan and can provide more detailed pictures of the heart and blood vessels. The MRI can show the heart from many different angles and provide information on its size as well as the functioning of its chambers, the thickness of the heart walls, and the presence of any congenital defects. It can also give detailed views of blood vessels and even detect clots in the blood. However, an MRI cannot show calcium deposits as well as an ordinary X-ray or CT scan can.

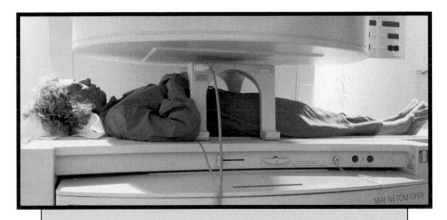

This woman is undergoing an MRI, which doesn't involve any radiation exposure as other imaging tests do, so there are no health risks involved.

ECHOCARDIOGRAPHY

Echocardiography is a diagnostic technique that uses ultrasound (sounds too high-pitched for humans to hear) to produce images of structures inside the body. The concept is much like the way bats use echolocation to find their way in the dark. In echocardiography, ultrasound waves are sent into the body and reflected (echoed) back from structures inside the body. These ultrasounds are received by a small recording instrument, called the transducer, placed on the chest. As the transducer moves over the target area, the "echos" are then translated by a computer and turned into a detailed computer image, which can be recorded on videotape or printed on paper. The echocardiogram (image) shows detailed pictures of the heart chambers, heart valves, and major blood vessels running to and from the heart. It can provide a wealth of information about the health of the heart and blood vessels, including the heart's size, the heart's pumping abilities, damage to the heart muscle, structural abnormalities, type and severity of valve problems, and blood-flow problems.

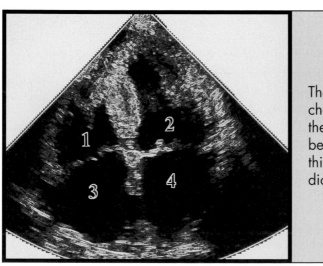

The four chambers of the heart can be seen in this echocardiogram.

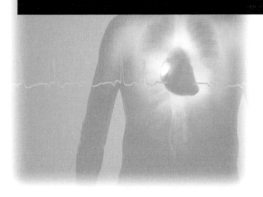

MENDING BROKEN HEARTS

A STORY ABOUT JANET AND HER DAD, DAN

Janet was really excited about starting her fresh-man year at a local college. This would be the first time she would be living away from home. She and her dad, Dan, spent all morning loading up the van with all her belongings. There was so much stuff, her father joked that it was lucky Janet wasn't taking the bed, too.

After they arrived at the college, Janet noticed that her dad was sweating a lot and pulling at his collar, like he was a little short of breath. She figured that he was probably just uncomfortable because it was a really hot day. Janet needed to fill out a few more forms at the Registrar's Office before they could unload the van. After waiting about twenty minutes in line, Janet noticed that her dad looked pale and was a little wobbly on his feet. Then he suddenly grabbed his arm and dropped to the floor.

Janet screamed and tried desperately to get her father to "wake up." She realized that he was having a heart attack. She remembered learning about the signs of a heart attack in health class back in high school. But Janet was so scared, she didn't know what to do. Soon a crowd of people stood around them, and someone yelled to call an ambulance. An office worker named Sara fought her way through the crowd and told Janet that she knew cardiopulmonary resuscitation (CPR). Sara leaned over Dan and found that he was not breathing. Then she performed CPR for about five minutes until the ambulance came.

A paramedic took over for Sara while another one examined Dan. The paramedics told the people to step back so they could do their job. Then one of the paramedics used a defibrillator on Dan to start his heart beating again. It worked, and the paramedics told Sara that thanks to her quick response, Dan now had another chance at life.

IN CASE OF AN EMERGENCY

Would you know what to do in an emergency? When we're young, we are usually taught a simple yet important rule: in case of an emergency, call 9-1-1! That's really good advice, and it could someday save a life. For example, when someone is having a heart attack, calling 9-1-1 right away is important. The sooner the person gets help, the better the chance for survival. But sometimes even that may not be quick enough. If the heart stops pumping, the brain cells will be starved. The victim may suffer brain damage or even die in just a few minutes. Many people are

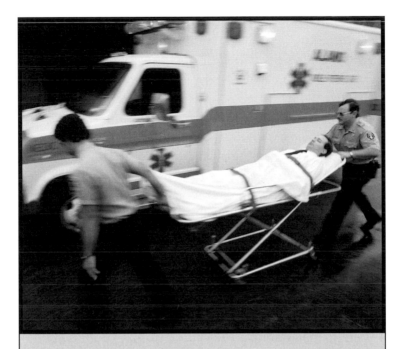

It is crucial that paramedics get to the scene as soon as possible when someone has a heart attack. Time is one of the most important factors in saving a person's life.

learning how to do CPR, which is a way to keep a heart attack victim alive until the ambulance comes. Anyone can learn how to do CPR. (Sara learned how to do it so she could help her children in case of an emergency.) It doesn't need any special machines or equipment. A person who has been trained in this lifesaving technique presses on the victim's chest to keep the heart pumping and breathes into the victim's mouth to send air into the lungs.

Surviving a heart attack is only half the battle. The next step is to find out how seriously the heart was damaged. Doctors will use various diagnostic techniques, dis-

WHAT A SHOCK!

We're all familiar with that scene on TV or in the movies—the patient's heart stops beating, so the doctor in the emergency room grabs two paddles, places them on top of the person's chest, and yells "Clear!" The defibrillator sends out a powerful shock that will hopefully kick-start the heart into beating again. After a few jolts, the heart is working in a normal rhythm, and the patient "comes back to life."

Defibrillators are valuable lifesaving devices. Emergency personnel usually have them on hand when responding to a call for help. Now portable defibrillators can be found in a number of public places such as sports stadiums, airport terminals, theaters, shopping malls, and even airplanes. Having them on the scene when an emergency occurs makes it possible to treat the victim quickly, before it's too late.

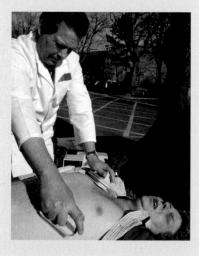

A paramedic resuscitates a man with a portable defibrillator.

cussed in the previous chapter, to determine the severity of the condition before they can choose appropriate treatment. Depending on the situation, treatment may be as simple as taking heart medication, or the condition may be so serious that heart surgery may be needed. In some cases, the heart damage is too severe to be fixed, and a heart transplant is the only hope for survival.

HEART MEDICATIONS

There is no magic pill to cure heart disease, but there are more than one hundred different medications available to treat the symptoms of people with cardiovascular problems. In the hospital, doctors can inject drugs shortly after a heart attack to dissolve blood clots in the coronary arteries. A number of drugs can help to relieve angina. A well-known one, nitroglycerin, is so effective that it can stop angina pain within two minutes. Nitroglycerin comes in tablets that dissolve when placed under the tongue. Once the drug gets into the bloodstream, it works by expanding the coronary arteries, allowing blood to flow past the fatty buildup.

Some other medications that are used to help ease angina are called beta-blockers and calcium channel blockers. Beta-blockers help to slow the heart rate and lessen the need for oxygen so that the heart doesn't have to work as hard. Calcium channel blockers work in a similar way as beta-blockers, and they also widen the coronary arteries. Both types of drugs also help to lower high blood pressure, as do dozens of others. Some work by stimulating the kidneys to get rid of excess water, lightening the load on the heart.

Medications are also available to help lower cholesterol levels in the blood, control the heartbeat rhythm, and help to clear the fatty plaques out of arteries. There are even drugs that can help seal up the hole in the heart septum of some newborn babies.

Many doctors recommend taking half an aspirin every day to reduce the chance of a heart attack. Aspirin makes the blood platelets less likely to stick together and produce blood clots in coronary arteries. It also reduces inflammation. These drug actions make aspirin effective in preventing both heart attacks and strokes that are due to plugging of a brain artery by a clot. But it can somewhat increase the danger of the less common kind of stroke, which is due to the bursting of a weak spot in an artery. Aspirin can also be effective as a first-aid treatment for a heart attack. Chewing an aspirin tablet within thirty minutes after the attack has started can help prevent severe damage to the heart muscle. (Chewing gets the drug absorbed into the body faster than just swallowing it whole.)

GYPSY REMEDY

In 1775, Dr. William Withering was one of the most successful doctors in England, and patients flocked to his office in Birmingham. He had also written a huge book on the plants of Great Britain and how they are used in medicine. But he could not suggest a cure for one patient, a man who was suffering from severe congestive heart failure. So the man consulted another "expert," an old gypsy woman who was known for her secret herbal remedies. After drinking the old gypsy's herbal tea, the patient was delighted to find that his hugely swollen ankles were soon back to normal, he could breathe more easily, and he had more energy.

Hearing about this amazing recovery, Dr. Withering tracked down the old gypsy and bargained with

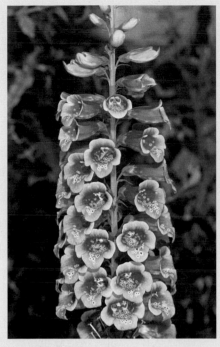

Digitalis
purpurea

her for the recipe of her herbal tea. It was a mixture
of more than twenty different herbs, but with his vast
knowledge of botany, the doctor soon figured out
that the active herb was purple foxglove, *Digitalis
purpurea*. Extracts of this popular garden plant had
long been used as a poison. Dr. Withering began giving his heart patients tiny doses of digitalis, too small
to be harmful. It worked so well that ten years later,
he published a scientific paper on its medical uses.
Today, forms of digitalis are still among the most
effective drugs for people with congestive heart failure. They increase the strength of the heart's contractions and slow down the heart rate.

ARTIFICIAL PACEMAKER

If a heart rhythm becomes too slow or "skips a beat," a person's natural pacemaker may be faulty. Medication may be able to help the heartbeat get back on track, but sometimes it may not be enough. Then the person may need to have an *artificial* pacemaker implanted.

An artificial pacemaker is a small, battery-operated device that is designed to "sense" if there's a problem in the heart rhythm, and if needed, it produces electrical signals to keep the heart beating regularly and at a suitable pace. The device, also called a generator, is implanted under the skin in the upper chest. It is connected to wires, called leads, which are attached to a large vein leading to the heart. The leads send out tiny bursts of electricity through the vein to the heart, signaling it to beat.

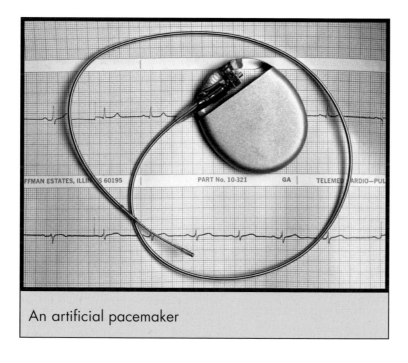

An artificial pacemaker

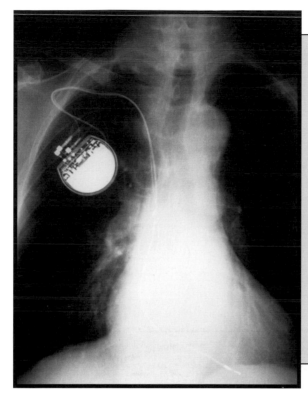

This is an X-ray of an artificial pacemaker implanted in the upper chest.

Originally, the artificial pacemaker was designed strictly to keep the heart beating normally when it becomes too slow or skips a beat. Now, modern pacemakers work more like a real heart—they not only keep the heart beating regularly, but they can also speed up or slow down the heart according to the activity level. Over 100,000 Americans are implanted with pacemakers every year.

A newer device, the implantable cardioverter defibrillator (ICD), acts like an artificial pacemaker when the heartbeat is too slow or irregular. If the heart begins to beat so fast that it cannot pump effectively, the device acts as a defibrillator, delivering a jolt of electricity to shock the heart back into a more normal rhythm. In a study reported in 2003, more than six hundred patients who had had a heart attack or were suffering from heart failure had 30 percent fewer deaths over a period of two years after they were given an ICD, compared with a similar group who received only medical treatments. ICDs are still very expensive though—up to $50,000 to implant one—and patients say that their lifesaving shocks feel like the kick of a mule.

BALLOON ANGIOPLASTY

Most blocked arteries can be treated with medication and lifestyle changes. But if the blockage is too severe, or if several arteries are blocked, surgery may be necessary. The doctor may have to perform a balloon angioplasty to clear out the blocked artery. In this procedure, a catheter with a tiny balloon at the tip is slipped through the blood vessel into the clogged area. The balloon is inflated, pushing out the artery walls so that blood can flow freely. After the artery is cleared, the balloon is deflated and the catheter is removed. Often this procedure involves inserting a stent in the artery. A stent is a wire-mesh tube that helps to keep the artery open. However, for as many as a third of those who have an angioplasty, the artery may become narrowed or blocked again within six months. This is most likely to occur in people with diabetes, and in those who continue their bad habits such as smoking, eating fatty foods, and staying inactive. If the artery does close up again, the doctor will need to perform a second angioplasty. Researchers are now testing new kinds of stents with a nonstick coating. They slowly release tiny amounts of drugs that prevent cells from growing over the stent.

Laser angioplasty is sometimes used either together with balloon angioplasty or by itself. In this procedure, a catheter with a laser at its tip is inserted. When it reaches the blockage, the laser sends out high-energy light pulses that vaporize the plaque.

OPEN-HEART SURGERY

If too much of the artery is blocked, and it cannot simply be "cleaned out," the doctor may have to perform open-heart surgery. Generally, "open-heart surgery" refers to an operation in which the heart and blood vessels are worked on, and a heart-lung machine is used. During surgery, doctors stop the heart with medications and use a heart-lung machine, commonly called the "pump." The heart-lung machine is an electronic device that takes over the work of these organs, pumping oxygen-rich blood into the body during surgery. Tubes inserted into blood vessels carry blood out of the body to the machine and then back again. This allows doctors to work more effectively on the heart while it is not moving. When surgery is completed, the surgeon restarts the heart, and the pump is removed so that the heart and lungs can get back to working on their own again.

Bypass Surgery

The most common type of heart surgery performed in the United States is coronary artery bypass graft, or CABG (pronounced "cabbage") surgery, more commonly known as bypass surgery. In this surgical procedure, instead of unblocking the clogged artery, the surgeon reconstructs the network of arteries to detour around, or bypass, the one that's blocked. This is done by taking a piece of a long vein from the patient's leg, or an artery from inside the chest cavity, and then sewing one end to the aorta—the large artery leaving the heart. By attaching (grafting) the other end of the vein to the coronary artery beyond the blocked area, the surgeon creates a new route for blood to flow to the heart muscle, bringing in the important oxygen and nutrients that the heart needs to work effectively. Depending on how many arteries are blocked, a person may need more than one bypass. You may have heard people talk about a "triple bypass" or a "quadruple bypass." These

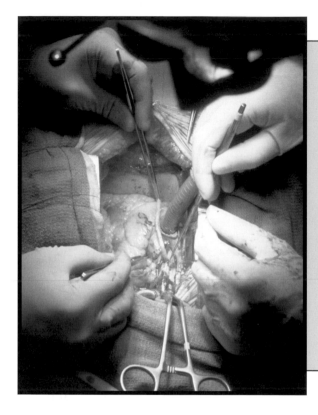

This is a picture of the heart during a coronary bypass operation.

are surgeries that involve rerouting three or four blocked arteries.

Traditionally, a heart-lung machine is used in bypass surgeries. However, there have been concerns about the pump causing problems such as inflammation of the lungs, heart, and other organs, as well as memory loss and even stroke. This has led to an increasing number of bypass surgeries that are being performed "off pump"—while the heart is beating. The surgeon uses a device that stabilizes the heart. The area where the surgeon is working is fairly still, but the rest of the heart is still beating. Doctors have found that in some patients, off-pump bypass surgery has more benefits than traditional bypass surgery. These benefits include quicker recovery, shorter hospital stay, less chance for memory loss or stroke, less blood loss, and better survival rate.

Off-pump bypass surgery is not yet standard practice. Most bypasses still use a heart-lung machine. Some medical experts hope that off-pump surgeries will become increasingly common. However, not all patients make good candidates for off-pump bypass surgery, especially those patients with seriously weakened hearts, high-risk patients, and patients with severely narrowed arteries.

Heart-Valve Repairs

Surgeons may also perform heart surgery to repair or replace damaged heart valves. Heart-valve problems may be present at birth, may be caused by a disease such as rheumatic fever, or may be the result of aging. Certain kinds of damage or defects can be repaired. Others cannot be repaired, and the valves must be replaced. There are

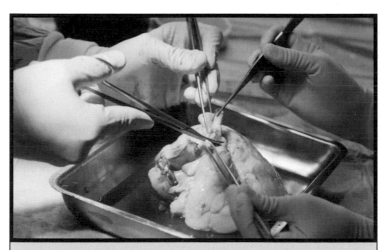

Here, a heart is being prepared at an organ bank. The valves are being removed in order to replace a patient's damaged valve.

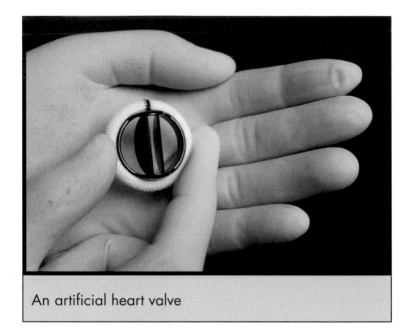

An artificial heart valve

several kinds of replacement heart valves. Surgeons may use valves from pigs' hearts, valves made from the pericardium of cows, human valves taken from a person who died, or artificial heart valves. Artificial valves are made of plastic or metal. They are much more durable, but they can cause blood clots. So people who receive artificial valves must take anticoagulant (anticlotting) drugs for the rest of their lives.

Most valve problems involve the mitral valve, the one that controls blood flow from the left atrium to the left ventricle. That's because blood flows through the mitral valve with a much greater force than through the other heart valves. So when the mitral valve slams shut, it has to hold back all that tremendous pressure. As a result, this valve may eventually weaken until it can no longer function effectively.

The most common mitral valve problem is actually a congenital condition called *mitral valve prolapse*. It affects about 3 to 5 percent of the adult population. In this condition, the valve has more tissue than it needs to snap shut. Instead of lying flat as the valve closes, the tissue bulges backward into the left atrium (prolapses), allowing some blood to flow back into the heart's upper chamber.

HEART TRANSPLANTS

If the heart is so damaged that it can't be repaired, a heart transplant may be suggested. This is an operation in which the damaged heart is removed and replaced with a healthy one from someone who has just died. (Donor hearts come from people who are brain-dead but have healthy, beating hearts. Many heart donors are victims who die in car accidents.) The demand for hearts is much greater than the supply. More than 4,000 patients are on the national waiting list for heart transplants, but only about 2,200 donor hearts become available every year. How much time a person has to wait depends on a number of factors, including the blood type, a size match between the donor and recipient, and the severity of the patient's medical condition. Depending on the situation, the wait may be only a few weeks, or it may take years to find a donor. Many people die before their name comes up on the list.

When a heart donor match is found, time is critical. A healthy heart cannot exist outside a person's body for more than four hours. Once the heart is removed, it is stored in a special cold solution. The medical team then quickly ships the heart to the location of the recipient. The heart transplant begins shortly thereafter.

The first heart transplant was performed in 1967 by Dr. Christiaan Barnard in South Africa. However, early heart transplants were not successful, because, at the time, doctors did not realize that the body would attack the "foreign" cells in the new heart. This reaction is known as rejection. Now that doctors are more familiar with how the immune system works, survival rates have greatly

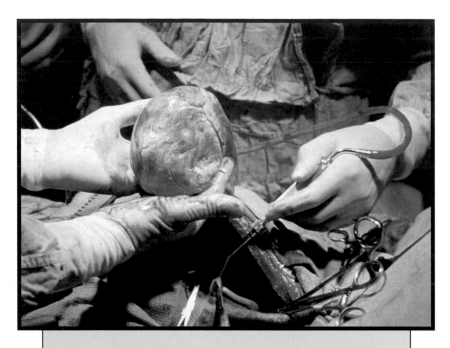

This is one of the original heart transplant surgeries being performed in 1968. The new heart is being placed into the forty-eight-year-old recipient's chest.

improved. Powerful drugs that weaken the immune system, called *immunosuppressants*, must be taken for the rest of the patient's life to prevent rejection after the heart transplant. However, people who take them are more vulnerable to infection, and they can die from a normally harmless illness.

Heart transplants have given thousands of people another chance at life. An estimated 85 percent survive one year after the transplant, about 77 percent survive three years after, 71 percent survive five years after the operation, and 50 percent survive ten years after.

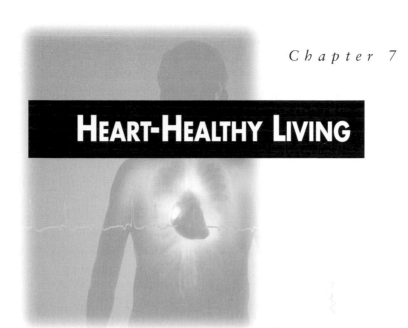

Chapter 7

HEART-HEALTHY LIVING

JERRY'S STORY

At six feet one (185 cm), 260 pounds (118 kg), Jerry Matthews knew that he should lose some weight. He had heard all the health warnings. But when it came to some of his favorite foods—pizza, cheeseburgers, fried chicken, and mashed potatoes loaded with butter—he just couldn't resist. It didn't help that he never exercised, either. As a computer technician, Jerry spent a lot of time sitting during the day, and by the time he'd get home from work, he would plop down on the couch and watch TV. But at twenty-nine years old, Jerry wasn't too concerned about his health. I'm still young, he figured. There's time.

A few days before Jerry turned thirty, he went to the doctor's office for a routine physical. He knew he wasn't in the best shape, but still, he was surprised when he found out the results of his blood test. He had a total cholesterol level of 290, which is 90 points beyond the normal range. If Jerry didn't lower his cholesterol level significantly, he could have a heart attack at an early age. The doctor told Jerry that he needed to change to a healthier lifestyle, and that meant exercise and cutting down on fatty foods.

Over the next six months, Jerry got into a vigorous exercise program, and he ate healthy foods (although he splurged once in a while). He ate less meat and more fish and chicken (baked not fried!). He also cut down on his portions. Jerry managed to lose about forty pounds, and he felt a lot better about himself. And his cholesterol dropped forty-five points! The doctor was impressed with Jerry's progress and told him that if he continues this heart-healthy lifestyle, his cholesterol could soon fall into the normal range.

There are some risk factors we can't control—we can't change our parents or whether we're male or female or how old we are. Does that mean that there's no hope? That a person with these kinds of risk factors is just a ticking time bomb waiting to go off? Not at all. There are many things that people can do to reduce their risks for heart disease. They need to eliminate the risk factors that they *can* control, such as smoking, overeating, and being inactive. For most people, heart problems do not develop until middle age, but as we have learned, it's never too early to start thinking heart-smart.

EAT HEALTHY

Developing healthy eating habits is one of the most important ways to prevent heart disease. It can help to reduce three important risk factors: high blood cholesterol, high

REALLY BAD FATS

Oils that contain large amounts of unsaturated fats
may spoil if they are exposed to the oxygen in the
air. Food manufacturers often treat vegetable oils
with hydrogen, which turns them into partly saturated forms that don't spoil when exposed to oxygen.
Cookies, crackers, and other foods made with these
"partially hydrogenated" oils can be kept on the
shelf without refrigeration for much longer times.
Recent studies suggest, however, that hydrogen-
treated "trans fats" are even worse for people's heart
health than naturally saturated fats are. Food manufacturers are catching on, and processed foods
labeled "No Trans Fats" are starting to appear on
grocery shelves.

blood pressure, and excess body weight. Part of healthy
eating is choosing foods that are low in saturated fat and
cholesterol. Saturated fat is usually solid at room temperature. It is found in fatty meats, dairy products, coconut oil,
and palm and palm kernel oil, and it tends to raise cholesterol levels in the blood. It is better to eat foods that contain unsaturated fats, which are usually liquid at room
temperature and come mainly from plant sources, such as
olive oil, corn oil, canola oil, and safflower oil. Seeds and
nuts also contain unsaturated fats. These are better choices
than foods that are high in saturated fat. Product labels
usually break down the fat content into saturated,
monounsaturated, and polyunsaturated fats.

Would you be able to make the right choices? Which
food is loaded with saturated fat—a doughnut or a bagel?
The answer is a doughnut. But if the bagel is smeared with

cream cheese, then it becomes an unhealthy choice—unless the cream cheese is low-fat or fat-free. Many low-fat or no-fat products are available these days that provide good alternatives to less-healthy foods.

WHICH DIET IS BEST?

For years, health experts have been telling us that the best way to lose weight is to reduce fats in our diet and to eat complex carbohydrates (such as breads, whole-grain rice, and yams), but not refined sugars (such as those in candy bars, cookies, and ice cream). So it came as a shock when Dr. Robert Atkins presented a completely different kind of diet plan. In fact, it was exactly the opposite of what was generally accepted. The Atkins Diet, as it is popularly known, is a plan that is low in carbohydrates but high in fat and protein. People who follow this diet can eat as much cheese, steak, and low-carb ice cream as they want and still lose weight. Critics say this plan is ridiculous. However, some studies have shown that people on the Atkins Diet may lose more weight than those on the standard low-fat diets without increasing cholesterol levels, and they do it faster. Health experts find the results "hard to believe."

The Atkins Diet remains controversial. Researchers continue to conduct studies so they can figure out why this and other low-carb, high-fat, high-protein diets actually work. Interestingly, despite all the research and technology we have today, scientists are still arguing about what makes up a healthy diet.

Carbohydrates, and especially refined sugars, can also contribute to fat problems. Body cells can turn sugars into fats. For some people, eating too much sugar causes the triglyceride level in the blood to rise. Eating too many calories from any kind of food can also result in obesity, which could lead to diabetes, a disease that greatly increases the risk of heart attacks.

High-fiber foods are good for the heart, though. Fiber helps to move digestion along. It also lowers blood cholesterol and triglyceride levels. Good sources of fiber are fruits (such as apples), vegetables (such as beans and spinach), and whole-grain breads and cereals.

The U.S. Food Guide Pyramid can help people choose what foods they should eat and how much. This is a special diagram that places the foods we eat into five main groups. The amounts that a person should eat each day get smaller as you move from the foods at the bottom of the

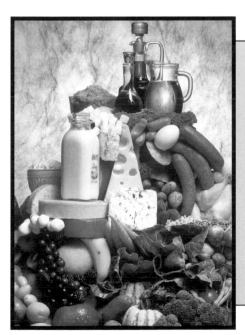

This is the U.S. Food Guide Pyramid showing the foods that each of the five groups represents. The amount that a person should eat becomes smaller as you move from the bottom to the top.

GOOD HEART FOODS

You may have heard that fish is good brain food, but it's good for your heart, too. In fact, fish may actually help reduce the risk of heart disease. Researchers have found that oily fish such as salmon, tuna, and sardines contain large amounts of omega-3 fatty acids, which are a form of polyunsaturated fats that helps to lower triglycerides and raise HDL ("good" cholesterol) when eaten as part of a heart-healthy diet. Health experts recommend that people eat fish (especially oily fish) at least twice a week. Eskimos, who eat a diet high in oily fish, have a very low heart-attack rate.

Nuts are good for your heart, too. Peanuts, peanut butter, and peanut oil are high in monounsaturated fats, and studies have shown that they help to lower both cholesterol and triglycerides. Walnuts are high in polyunsaturated fats and are an excellent source of omega-3 fatty acids, both of which help to reduce the risk of heart disease. Other nuts can also help. But don't overdo it! Nuts are high in calories, and up to 80 to 90 percent of those calories are fats; so eating too many nuts can lead to weight gain—raising the heart-disease risk. Small amounts are all you need: eating 1 ounce (28 g) of nuts a day, at least five days a week, can reduce the risk of heart disease by 25 to 50 percent.

Another good-for-the-heart food may surprise you: chocolate! Chemicals in dark chocolate may help prevent heart disease in several different ways.

They help to prevent LDL cholesterol from forming plaques in artery walls, they relax blood vessels and help to prevent high blood pressure, and they make blood platelets less likely to stick together and form clots that could lead to a heart attack or stroke. But like nuts, chocolate is high in calories—so don't eat too much!

To be most effective, all these foods should be eaten as part of a heart-healthy diet.

pyramid to those at the top. Starting at the bottom and moving upward, the five groups include: (1) the bread, cereal, rice, and pasta group; (2) the fruits and vegetables group; (3) the milk, yogurt, and cheese group; (4) the meat, poultry, fish, dry beans, eggs, and nuts group; and (5) the fats, oils, and sweets group.

In general, nutrition experts recommend that two-thirds of the diet should come from plant foods—fruits, vegetables, grains, and legumes (beans). The other third should come from animal foods—meat, fish, poultry, and dairy products. The American Heart Association Eating Plan for Healthy Americans, released in 2000 and revised in 2004, provides some helpful guidelines to follow:

- Watch your portion sizes and limit total calories to the amount needed for a healthy weight.

- Eat at least five servings of fruits and vegetables per day.

- Eat at least six servings of grain products per day; choose whole grains over processed grains.

- Eat fish at least two times a week.

- Include fat-free and low-fat milk products, legumes, skinless poultry, and lean meats.

- Choose monounsaturated and polyunsaturated fats and oils, such as olive, canola, peanut, and safflower oils and margarines.

- Limit foods high in saturated fats and/or cholesterol, such as whole milk products, fatty meats, and egg yolks. Avoid trans fats, found in partially hydrogenated vegetable oils.

- Limit foods high in calories or low in nutrition, such as soft drinks and candy.

- Limit the intake of salt or sodium to no more than 1 teaspoon or less than 2,300 mg of sodium per day.

More details can be found on the website at http://www.everydaychoices.org.

Not every meal has to meet all these guidelines, but they should apply to a person's overall eating routine. According to health experts, reducing cholesterol levels alone could cut down heart disease deaths by 20 to 30 percent.

Research studies suggest that antioxidants, which include beta-carotene and vitamins C and E, might help to prevent heart disease. Antioxidants are found mainly in fruits and vegetables, especially the brightly colored ones. They help to prevent damaging reactions of oxygen with body chemicals that produce very reactive substances called *free radicals*. Free radicals can cause changes in fatty acids and LDL cholesterol in the blood. These changes may make it easier for body cells to absorb fatty acids and LDLs, which can lead to plaque buildup that blocks the arteries. Antioxidants may reduce the risk of heart disease by slowing down the oxidative process. Some foods that are rich in antioxidants are collard greens, broccoli, spinach, tomatoes, potatoes, strawberries, oranges, grapefruit, vegetable oils (and products made with them), wheat germ, and nuts.

For some people, eating healthy may not be enough to reduce their high cholesterol level or high blood pressure. In that case, they will have to take medication to keep their cholesterol and blood pressure at normal levels. But it is important to stay on a heart-healthy diet as well.

STAY ACTIVE

Staying physically fit is another good way to prevent heart disease. People who are couch potatoes may increase a number of risk factors, including obesity, high blood pressure, high triglycerides, a low level of HDL, and diabetes. Exercise doesn't have to consist of intense workouts every day of the week. In fact, simply going on fast-paced walks for thirty minutes or more on most days of the week can reduce the risk for heart disease. Young people who devel-

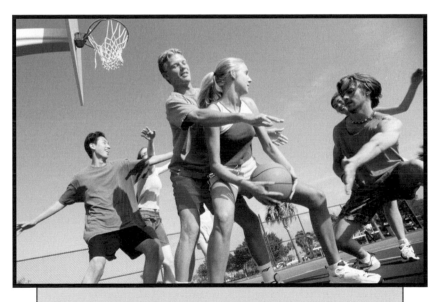

Getting involved in sports activities is a great way to stay physically fit, and it's a lot of fun, too.

op the habit of being active are more likely to stay active as they grow into adults.

Exercise can provide benefits in a number of ways:

- It tones up the heart, lungs, and blood vessels and makes the circulation of blood throughout the body more effective.

- It helps to keep body weight down.

- It stimulates the production of HDLs, and lowers the levels of LDLs.

- It helps to reduce tension and stress.

- It lowers the blood-sugar level and helps to control diabetes.

- It stimulates the coronary artery blood vessels to branch and grow, which provides the heart with extra blood supply to help the heart work more effectively. This also provides many alternative routes to the heart muscle if one artery should happen to be blocked.

DON'T SMOKE

Of all the risk factors, smoking is one of the easiest to avoid. If you don't smoke, it's a good idea not to start. If you already do smoke, then try to quit. The nicotine in cigarette smoke is not only harmful, but it is also addictive. Once you start smoking, your body starts to "crave" this harmful chemical, which makes it much harder to stop. When the body isn't getting its usual dose of chemicals, the smoker may feel restless and irritable, hungry, headachy, and depressed. These are withdrawal symptoms. Anybody who wants to quit smoking can talk to a doctor to find out the best way to do it with the least possible withdrawal symptoms. Products are available to help people quit, such as nicotine patches and nicotine gum. Some people can even quit cold turkey—they stop smoking without the help of any devices. Eventually, the need for nicotine goes away. One year after a smoker quits, his or her risk of heart disease is half that of a smoker's. After ten years, the risk is about the same as that of a nonsmoker.

MANAGE DIABETES

People who have diabetes can reduce their risk for heart disease by keeping their blood-sugar levels under control. First of all, it is very important to eat a well-balanced, low-fat diet, and to keep a healthy weight. Obesity is a serious risk factor for type 2 diabetes. At least 80 percent of people with diabetes weigh 20 percent or more than they should. Just losing half of this excess weight is enough to prevent diabetes.

Exercise is also important in keeping diabetes under control. When you exercise, sugar is burned for energy, and the blood-glucose level decreases. Exercise also burns up food materials that might otherwise be stored in the body as fat. This helps to avoid obesity, which can make diabetes symptoms worse.

Monitoring glucose is an important part of managing diabetes. People with diabetes need to check their blood glucose levels several times a day to see how well their condition is being controlled. This helps to give a better idea of how much insulin is needed. Blood glucose monitors are devices that can measure blood-sugar levels in a matter of minutes. Using a monitor regularly helps you to figure out how much insulin you need.

Blood sugar is usually tested by pricking a finger or earlobe and placing a drop of blood into a small portable machine that provides a digital readout of blood-sugar levels. Glucose monitoring is very important because it helps to avoid serious problems that may develop.

REDUCE STRESS

Everybody gets stressed out from time to time, but how people deal with the stress may determine their risk for heart disease. Different people handle stress differently—and studies have found that certain personality traits seem to contribute to the development of heart problems. These are impatience, hostility, and intense anger.

Does waiting in line make you feel like you are wasting time? Does it make you annoyed and irritable? If someone cuts in front of you, do you blow up in anger, yelling or even getting physical? If so, you may be setting yourself up for a heart attack someday. A recent study conducted at Northwestern University showed that young adults who have hostile and impatient personalities are more likely to develop high blood pressure by their forties—putting them at a greater risk for developing heart disease.

People who are impatient and hostile as kids will probably be that way as adults. But the situation is not hopeless. People can learn to be more easygoing and take things in stride. They can learn not to let little things bother them—especially things they cannot do anything about. Learning to deal with anger and stress when you are young can greatly reduce your risk for a heart attack when you get older.

There are a number of things that people can do to help them deal with stressful situations better, without getting too stressed out. They can help you in everyday life, too.

First, when you are faced with a stressful situation, take a deep breath. Slowly inhale through your nose and then slowly exhale. Deep breathing can actually lower your blood pressure and pulse rate.

Exercise is a great way to work off any "nervous energy." It can also put you in a good mood. When you exercise, your brain produces chemicals called *endorphins*, which work to make you feel happy. The more you exercise, the more endorphins your body makes. It doesn't take much time—even a twenty-minute walk a few times a week can have health and relaxation benefits. Also, doing exercises specifically to relax your muscles can be very helpful. The parts of the body that experience the most tension are the neck, the shoulders, the jaw, and the back.

Meditation is also helpful in lowering the heart rate, blood pressure, and stress-hormone level. Using your imagination to create soothing scenery in your mind can also help you to relax.

Eat a healthy diet and don't skip meals. This can help you to feel your best, and it will keep you from running out of energy during the day. Also, chewing can actually release tension in your jaw muscles.

Get a good night's sleep. This will allow you to feel refreshed when you wake up, and ready to tackle the day.

Pets can be good stress-relievers. Studies have shown that pet owners have lower blood pressure than those without pets. Talking to your pets keeps you from thinking about yourself and all of the things you need to do.

Set aside some time in the day to talk with your family to develop better communication between all members.

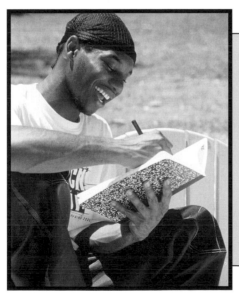

Write down your problems in a journal. This can help you sort them out and make them more manageable and understandable.

Also, tape TV shows to watch when it is more convenient, so you can spend some quality time with your family.

Talk to someone about your problems, whether it be a good friend, a family member, or a counselor. Keeping your anger and frustration to yourself can be very unhealthy, both emotionally and physically.

Worrying about everything is a waste of energy. Can you control what you're worrying about? If not, then don't waste your time.

Procrastinating can be very stressful. When you put things off, you spend all your time worrying about it. But when a job is done right away, there's no more reason to get all worked up over it.

Lower your standards. The need for perfection can cause a lot of unnecessary stress. Nobody's perfect.

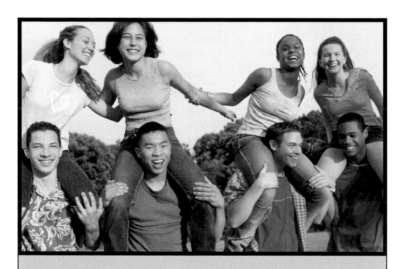

One of the best ways to handle stress is a good sense of humor. Laughter is really the best medicine. Research has shown that laughing inhibits stress hormones, and a good sense of humor helps to keep a person's stress level down.

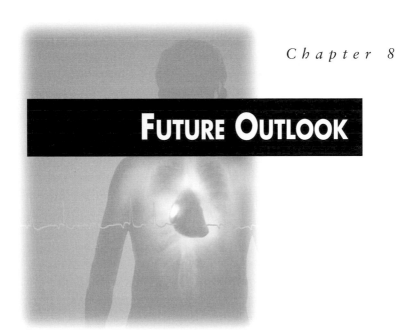

Chapter 8

FUTURE OUTLOOK

BARNEY CLARK'S STORY

In 1982, sixty-one-year-old retired dentist Barney Clark made medical history—he became the first person to receive a permanent artificial heart. His heart had been progressively failing, probably as a result of a virus infection that had attacked the heart muscle. Clark was a bit older than the usual heart-transplant recipients, but he had a fighting spirit, which convinced the doctors to give him a chance. On December 2, 1982, Dr. William DeVries, a veteran of more than two hundred artificial heart operations on sheep and calves and twenty on human cadavers, implanted a complete artificial heart, the Jarvik 7, in his first living human patient.

The operation was a success. There were problems, however, some of which were caused by the heart itself. For instance, doctors had to perform a second operation two weeks later to replace a broken heart valve. One of the problems was actually corrected by the artificial heart. When Barney Clark developed fluid in his lungs, the doctors just adjusted the dials on his control unit, which decreased the amount of blood being pumped to the lungs by the right ventricle and increased the amount being pumped to the body by the left ventricle. Treating the problem with drugs would have taken hours or even days, but in fifteen minutes, the artificial heart had removed all the excess fluid from Clark's lungs.

Another problem was that the Jarvik 7 had to be connected by hoses to an outside power source. Clark could not move more than 6 feet (1.8 m) from the machine, which weighed 375 pounds (170 kg) and was as big as a large filing cabinet. As Barney Clark recovered from the operation and felt well enough to move around, he was constantly reminded that he was literally tied to this huge drive system. Needless to say, this was very inconvenient.

In the end, the operation was considered a relative "success." Barney Clark died 112 days after the operation. It wasn't the artificial heart that failed, but rather Clark's lungs and other body systems, which turned out to be in worse condition than the doctors had realized. Barney Clark was admired for his courage and good humor. After his death, the doctors studied the experience and analyzed the lessons they had learned. They realized that, in the future, a patient in stronger physical condition, with a better chance of survival, should be selected. The drive unit also needed to be more portable, one that could be carried around freely.

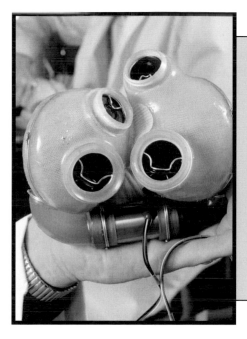

This is the Jarvik 7 artificial heart. Jarvik 7 was named after its inventor, Dr. Robert Jarvik, who remains active in the research and design of artificial heart devices.

Since then, Jarvik and other researchers have worked to improve artificial heart designs. One model currently being used, the AbioCor, is about the size of a grapefruit. A small, wearable battery transmits electric power to the implanted device through the skin, without any need for connecting tubes that could be a source of infection. Its two chambers supply blood to the lungs and to the organs of the body, pumping out as much as 2 gallons (8 L) of blood each minute. It is so quiet that a stethoscope is needed to listen to the heart sounds. In clinical trials, patients who received implanted AbioCor devices have survived for months; as of 2003, the record is seventeen months.

Meanwhile, mechanical devices have been used for more than two decades to assist rather than replace weakened hearts to keep people alive while they wait for a donor heart. Thousands of people have been kept alive using a mechanical pump called the *left ventricular assist device* (LVAD). This is a battery-operated pump that is surgically implanted in the left ventricle of the heart. It takes over the heart's pumping duties, sending oxygen-rich blood to the brain and the rest of the body. While the LVAD does the work, the heart gets to rest and heal. Generally, this device is used as a "bridge" to transplantation. But in November 2002, the FDA approved the LVAD as a form of treatment for people who do not qualify for heart transplants because of complications such as diabetes or other illnesses. This would give patients a chance to live longer than they would have under normal circumstances. In some cases, patients using the LVAD actually improve and no longer need heart transplants.

It seems unlikely that artificial hearts will be the ultimate solution to heart disease. How could enough artificial hearts be produced for the huge numbers of people whose hearts fail—and even if somehow they could, who would pay for them? Remember, in addition to the expense of producing an artificial heart and paying the surgeons and other highly trained members of the medical support staff to perform the operation of inserting it, each patient would then need careful follow-up care, including frequent checkups and a lifetime of taking medications to prevent strokes, treat infections, and so on.

ARE HEART TRANSPLANTS THE ANSWER?

What about heart transplants? Unfortunately, they are literally a dead end. For every person whose life is saved by a heart transplant, there must be someone else who died. Moreover, the heart donors must be people who died while their hearts were still healthy and strong, and the donor hearts must be removed quickly, before they start to decay.

Some medical experts have suggested using *xenotransplants*—the transplanting of organs from different species. Such operations have already been attempted. Back in

1964, a doctor in Mississippi transplanted a chimpanzee heart into a child whose own heart had severe defects. Since then, there have been attempts to transplant hearts from baboons, sheep, and pigs into human patients. All of these operations resulted in death of the transplant recipients, either during surgery or soon afterward as a result of rejection reactions. (If the body's defenses attack an organ transplant from another human, imagine how "foreign" they would find a transplant from a different species!) These medical experiments also sparked furious arguments about the ethics of the procedure, ranging from religious objections to accusations of cruelty to the human patient and to the animals that were sacrificed. (In the "Baby Fae" case in 1984, in which a baboon heart was transplanted into a baby girl, the hospital received 75 complaints about cruelty to Baby Fae, and 13,000 complaints about cruelty to the baboon.) Aside from the ethics of using hearts from chimpanzees or baboons, there are practical problems of supply—they are even scarcer than human heart donors.

The development of genetic engineering techniques, in which genes from one organism can be inserted into another, has given new life to the possibility of xenotransplants for ailing hearts. Pigs would probably be the donors of choice, since pigs' hearts are about the right size, and they are already slaughtered in huge numbers for food, leather, and other products, with few objections from animal lovers. Genetic engineers have been transferring some human genes to pigs and hope that transplants from these "humanized pigs" would be accepted by the body's defenses and would not cause rejection. Researchers are taking this work slowly, though, because there are some possible dangers. Viruses carried by the pigs might be transferred with a transplanted heart and cause an infectious disease or even cancer in the recipient. In addition, the lining of a pig's heart produces a substance that can lead to clotting of human blood. This is a trait that would have to be eliminated to make pig-human transplants safe.

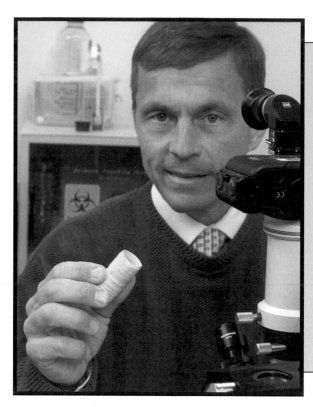

A research scientist shows a tube-shaped piece that was harvested from the bladder of a pig. The liver, stomach, and bladder of pigs have tissue that could potentially be used as replacement tissue in humans.

Meanwhile, researchers are working on another approach that would provide the ideal heart transplant: growing new hearts and other organs that are made of exact copies of the patient's own cells. Through techniques of tissue engineering, guided by the set of genetic instructions contained in each body cell, scientists hope to build a framework of the heart structure that would be filled out through the growth of all the specialized kinds of cells that formed the patient's original heart. Grown in a laboratory, in a tank filled with a solution containing nutrients and the proper chemicals to guide its development, the new heart could then be transplanted into the patient without any danger of rejection.

Stem cells, which have the potential to develop into almost every kind of cell in the body, could ultimately be used not only to grow new hearts for transplants, but also to repair damaged hearts right in the patient's body. The first successful experiments were done on mice. A research

WHAT ARE STEM CELLS?

The life of a human being starts when two microscopic cells—a sperm from the father and an egg cell from the mother—join to form a single cell that will develop into a new individual. That original cell divides again and again. At first, all the new cells are just the same as the original one (though a bit smaller), but soon the cells begin to divide into new, somewhat different kinds of cells. Some will go on to form skin, others eyes or muscles or nerves. Now the dividing cells are firmly committed to the tasks they will perform in the developing baby.

Scientists use the term "stem cells" for the cells at the earliest stages of development, which are still capable of developing into any kind of cell the body needs. In some tissues, such as the bone marrow where blood cells are formed, some stem cells remain even in adults. Such a stem cell may be called on to form red blood cells, which are doughnut-shaped disks, or white blood cells, which are like tiny animated blobs of jelly. In the laboratory, using different kinds of nutrients and growth factors, scientists have made bone-marrow stem cells divide into cells typical of different kinds of tissues—muscle or nerve cells, for example.

team at the New York Medical College in Valhalla, New York, injected stem cells from the bone marrow of a mouse into a damaged mouse heart. New heart muscle cells and new coronary blood vessels formed, and the heart regained some of its lost ability to pump blood.

Using a similar technique, human patients with congestive heart failure have been treated with stem cells taken from their bone marrow. The types of stem cells that influence the growth of heart muscle and bone vessels were specially selected for the transplants, which were injected directly into the heart muscle. In a study reported in 2004, ten patients who received the stem cell transplants in addition to coronary bypass surgery had a greater improvement in their heart function than ten patients who had only the bypass operation. Six months later, the hearts of the patients who had received stem-cell transplants were continuing to improve.

In 2005 an Argentine surgeon, Federico Benetti, announced that he had successfully treated ten human patients with congestive heart failure using stem cells from fetuses. The fetal stem cells produced their effect much more rapidly than adult stem cells used in earlier experiments. After a month, the pumping ability of the patients' hearts had increased by an average of 41 percent. In a six-minute test on a treadmill, the distance the patients could walk without having to stop increased 72 percent. "This brought about a dramatic change in the quality of life for most of the patients," Dr. Benetti said. "Some of them were in bed and could not walk before, but now they are leading a normal life."

RESEARCH CONTINUES

Growing new hearts for transplants and stimulating damaged hearts to repair themselves are still many years from becoming general medical practice. Meanwhile, research continues on developing better tests that can detect heart disease earlier, before too much damage has been done; better treatments with fewer side effects; and more effective ways to prevent heart attacks and other forms of heart disease.

The discovery that certain plaques are inflamed "hot spots," which may tear open after being attacked by the body's defenses, has suggested ways of finding and treating them. Do you recall what happens when you have an infected cut? The area around it gets red, swollen, painful, and hot. The usual imaging and scanning tests used to find plaque buildup in arteries are not able to pinpoint the location of the plaques most likely to cause trouble. But since inflammation generates heat, companies that make medical devices are working to build tiny heat-seeking sensors that can be guided into the arteries with a

ROBOTS IN THE OPERATING ROOM

Today's top heart surgeons are relying more and more on robot aids. These aren't independent robots, like R2D2 from *Star Wars*. Instead, they are remote-controlled robotic arms, equipped with cutters, grippers, and other tools, which the surgeon guides using hand controls and foot pedals. A tiny video camera that can be inserted into the heart through a 1/2-inch (1-cm) incision provides the surgeon with a 3-D view of the operating field that can be zoomed in for close-ups. Robotically assisted surgery has been used for bypass operations and the repair of defective heart valves. A recent study found that it is just as safe and effective as conventional surgery, and the patients recover more quickly because a much smaller incision is used.

ENGINEERING NEW
HEART-HEALTHY FOODS

Eggs, milk, and meat are an important part of the diet in the Western world. But these foods contain a lot of saturated fats and cholesterol, which are not very good for the heart and blood vessels. Oily fish such as salmon and sardines are high in the heart-healthy omega-3 fats, but many people do not like them. Others are worried about possible mercury contamination of ocean fish and the recent reports of PCBs and other cancer-causing industrial wastes that may be found in farm-grown salmon. Now genetic engineers are working on transferring genes for producing omega-3 fats to the livestock animals that produce eggs, milk, and meat. They have already bred a strain of mice that produce these "good fats," using a gene from a roundworm called *C. elegans* that converts other fatty acids to the omega-3 forms. The next step will be performing a similar feat in chickens, cows, and other livestock.

catheter, in much the same way that angiograms are performed now. The makers of MRI and CT scanners are also working on adapting those instruments to detect the troublesome plaques.

If doctors can find the plaques that may lead to heart attacks or stroke, what can they do about them? Late in 2003, heart researchers from the Cleveland Clinic announced that they had found an especially effective form of HDL and used it to treat patients with severe atherosclerosis. The active substance is a protein, which was found about twenty-five years before in a number of people in a village in northern Italy who had very low rates of heart disease. The Cleveland researchers said that this protein works like "Drano for the arteries"; in just six weeks of treatment, it removed more than 4 percent of the plaque deposits from their patients' arteries—a result about ten times as good as that for the best cholesterol-lowering drugs currently being used. Pfizer, a large drug company, has increased production of the protein for expanded tests.

Researchers are continuing to study large samples of heart-disease patients, looking for patterns that might reveal inherited differences from the general population. For example, it was announced in November 2003 that a mutation in a gene on chromosome 15, called MEF2A, doubles the risk of a heart attack in people who carry this particular form of the gene. This is a rather rare abnormality—most heart patients do not have this mutant gene. But learning about how it works can help to cast light on how heart disease can develop and may suggest ways to prevent it. The MEF2A gene helps to control the development of muscle tissue, including the muscles in the walls of the coronary arteries. It also helps to keep these muscles healthy and strong. People with the mutant form of the gene are believed to have a weakened inner lining of the coronary-artery walls, which makes them more likely to form plaque deposits. The researchers are counseling the members of the family in which the gene was discovered, advising those with the mutant gene to avoid smoking, eat a healthy diet, get plenty of exercise, and take medications if necessary to keep their cholesterol and blood pressure under control.

Heart-disease research has made huge strides in developing tests and treatments that are saving lives and improving the quality of life for people with heart disease. Meanwhile, medical experts say that diet, exercise, and other changes in lifestyle are the best ways to keep our hearts strong and healthy.

GLOSSARY

adrenaline—A hormone produced by the adrenal glands, which prepares the body for quick reactions to emergency situations. It raises the blood pressure and increases the heartbeat rate.

aneurysm—A weak spot in a blood vessel that may balloon out and burst.

angina pectoris (angina, for short)—Intense pressure or pain in the chest due to insufficient blood supply to the heart.

angiogram—X-rays showing the movement of an injected dye through blood vessels and heart chambers.

antioxidant—A substance that protects food or body chemicals from damage by oxygen.

aorta—The large artery leaving the heart that sends blood throughout the body.

arrhythmia—Unusual or irregular heartbeat, which may be either fast or slow.

artery (arteries *pl.*)—A blood vessel that carries blood away from the heart to any part of the body.

atherosclerosis—Hardening of the arteries due to the buildup of fatty deposits in the artery walls, to which minerals may be added; may also be called **arteriosclerosis**.

atrium (atria *pl.*)—The upper chamber of each side of the heart, which pumps blood into the ventricle.

balloon angioplasty—A procedure that surgically unclogs a blood vessel by inserting a balloon-tipped catheter (tube) to remove the plaque buildup.

blood clot—A gel-like, thickened lump formed by blood to close up a wound.

blood pressure—The pressure exerted by the blood on the walls of the blood vessels through which it is pumped.

blood vessels—Tubes that carry blood between the heart and all parts of the body.

bradycardia—A relatively slow heartbeat rate.

capillary—A tiny, thin-walled blood vessel connecting an artery with a vein.

cardiac arrest—Stopping of the heartbeat.

cardiac catheter—A long, flexible tube inserted into a blood vessel to reach the heart, used for diagnostic testing or procedures such as balloon angioplasty.

cardiologist—A doctor specializing in heart disease.

cardiomyopathy—An enlargement and weakening of the heart muscle, usually due to an infection or genetic mutation.

cardiopulmonary resuscitation (CPR)—A first-aid method that involves a combination of mouth-to-mouth breathing and pressing on the chest, used to keep a heart attack victim alive until medical help arrives.

cardiovascular disease—A condition involving the heart and blood vessels.

cardioverter—A device that senses when the heart begins to beat abnormally fast or fibrillates, and delivers an electric shock to bring it back into a more normal rhythm.

cholesterol—A fatty substance found in the plaque that clogs an artery. (It is also an important part of nerve cells.)

circulatory system—The heart and the network of blood vessels (arteries, veins, and capillaries) that deliver blood to all parts of the body.

congenital heart defects—Heart abnormalities that are present at birth.

congestion—A buildup of extra fluid in the tissues.

congestive heart failure—An illness in which the heart cannot pump enough blood, and as a result, body tissues fill with fluid; fluid in the lungs makes it hard to breathe; and the kidneys cannot remove all the poisons from the blood.

coronary arteries—Arteries that supply blood to the heart muscle.

coronary artery bypass graft (CABG) surgery—A surgical procedure that involves reconstructing the network of arteries to detour, or bypass, the one that is blocked.

coronary artery disease (CAD)—The most common form of heart disease, usually caused by atherosclerosis (a buildup of fatty plaques in one or more coronary arteries).

coronary thrombosis (coronary, for short)—A sudden blockage of a coronary artery by a blood clot, leading to a heart attack.

C-reactive protein (CRP)—A blood protein that is found in higher-than-normal amounts when inflammation is present in the body.

CT or CAT scan—A diagnostic tool in which tiny streams of X-rays are sent through the body at various angles to produce revealing pictures that are far clearer and more detailed than an ordinary X-ray image.

defibrillator—A device that delivers an electric shock to the heart muscle during fibrillation in order to restore the normal heart rhythm.

diabetes—A condition in which the hormone insulin is not produced or does not properly control the body's use and storage of glucose (sugar), resulting in abnormally high amounts of glucose in the blood; extra glucose may also spill over into the urine.

diastole—The relaxing part of the heartbeat cycle.

diastolic pressure—The blood pressure when the heart muscle is relaxed.

echocardiography—The use of high-frequency sound waves bounced off heart structures to show heart structures and their movements.

electrocardiograph (ECG or EKG)—A device that records the electrical activity of the heart. The record is called an electrocardiogram (also abbreviated ECG or EKG).

endorphins—Chemicals released in the body that send "happy messages" to the brain.

free radical—A highly reactive chemical that may be formed under the action of oxygen or radiation; free radicals can create changes in fatty acids and LDL cholesterol and may lead to heart disease.

heart attack—Sudden damage to the heart muscle that results when its blood supply is cut off.

heartbeat—A cycle of contraction and relaxation by the heart muscle as it pumps blood into the arteries.

heart murmur—A hissing sound heard between the sounds of the heartbeat.

heart valves—Structures that control the flow of blood in the heart; veins also contain valves.

high-density lipoproteins (HDLs)—"Good cholesterol"; fats in the blood that help carry cholesterol into the cells where it is needed.

hormones—Chemicals that help to control and coordinate body functions.

hypertension—High blood pressure.

immunosuppressant—A drug that prevents or reduces the normal immune system reactions.

infarction—An area in a tissue or organ in which cells have died when deprived of their blood supply.

left ventricular assist device (LVAD)—A battery-operated mechanical pump surgically implanted in the left ventricle of the heart. It takes over the heart's pumping duties while the heart gets to rest and heal; usually used as a "bridge" to a heart transplant.

lipids—Fatty chemicals, such as fats and cholesterol.

low-density lipoproteins (LDLs)—"Bad cholesterol"; fats in the blood that help to carry cholesterol into fatty deposits (plaques) in the artery walls.

magnetic resonance imaging (MRI)—A diagnostic tool that uses a strong magnetic field and radio waves that pass through the body to produce clear images of almost any organ in the body.

mitral valve prolapse—A birth defect in which the valve controlling the flow of blood from the left atrium to the left ventricle has extra tissue; instead of closing tightly, it bulges backward into the atrium and allows some blood to flow backward.

myocardial infarction—Heart attack; death of part of the heart muscle due to blockage of its blood supply.

myocardium—The heart muscle (cardiac muscle).

obesity—The condition of being extremely overweight.

pacemaker—A specialized part of the heart muscle that sets the regular heartbeat rhythm.

palpitations—An uncomfortable thumping feeling in the chest, created by a racing heartbeat.

pericardium—The sac enclosing the heart.

plaque—A fatty deposit in an artery wall.

platelets—Blood cell fragments that help blood to clot.

pulmonary circulation—The loops of blood vessels leading from the heart to the lungs and back again.

pulse—The rhythmic beating produced by contractions of the arteries that can be felt at various places where arteries pass close to the skin surface.

radioisotopes—Radioactive forms of an element.

rheumatic fever—An illness that may develop after a strep throat infection, causing thickening and scarring of the heart valves.

secondhand smoke—The smoke that is produced when someone else smokes tobacco.

septum—A muscular wall separating the chambers of the heart.

spasms—Sudden, uncontrolled contractions.

sphygmomanometer—An instrument used to measure blood pressure.

stem cells—Cells that have the potential to develop into any kinds of cells or tissues in the body.

stent—A wire-mesh tube that helps to keep an artery open.

stethoscope—An instrument used to listen to the heartbeat.

stress test—A recording of the heart's electrical activity made during exertion such as walking on a treadmill or pedaling a stationary bike.

stroke—A cutoff of the blood supply to a part of the brain, resulting in death of brain cells and loss of speech or other functions.

systemic circulation—The network of blood vessels carrying blood through all the parts of the body (except for those blood vessels going to and from the lungs).

systolic pressure—The blood pressure when the heart is contracting.

thrombus—A blood clot that forms inside a blood vessel.

trans fats—Fats or oils that have been treated with hydrogen to prevent spoiling.

triglycerides—Lipids found in foods that contain various fatty acids.

vein—A blood vessel that carries blood toward the heart.

ventricle—The thick-walled muscular lower chamber of each side of the heart, which pumps blood throughout the body.

ventricular fibrillation—A condition in which the heart quivers rapidly instead of contracting in a single unit, and does not pump blood.

xenotransplant—An organ or tissue transplanted into an individual of a different species.

RESOURCES

Organizations

American Heart Association
National Center
7272 Greenville Avenue
Dallas, TX 75231
Toll-free: 1-800-AHA-USA1 (1-800-242-8721)
Website: www.americanheart.org

American Society of Hypertension
148 Madison Avenue, Fifth Floor
New York, NY 10016
Phone: (212) 696-9099
Fax: (212) 696-0711
Website: www.ash-us.org/

Congenital Heart Information Network (C.H.I.N.)
1561 Clark Drive
Yardley, PA 19067
Phone: (215) 493-3068
Website: www.tchin.org/

Johns Hopkins Bayview Medical Center
Website: www.jhbmc.jhu.edu/cardiology/partnership/kids/kids
.topics.html
(Heart-healthy tips for children)

National Heart, Lung, and Blood Institute
National Institutes of Health
NHLBI Information Center

P.O. Box 30105
Bethesda, MD 20824-0105
Toll free: 1-800-575-WELL (1-800-575-9355)
Phone: (301) 592-8573
Website: www.nhlbi.nih.gov/

National Stroke Association
9707 East Easter Lane
Englewood, CO 80112
Toll-free: 1-800-STROKES (1-800-787-6537)
Phone: (303) 649-9299
Fax: (303) 649-1328
Website: www.stroke.org/

Books

American Heart Association. *Your Heart: An Owner's Manual.* Englewood Cliffs, NJ: Prentice Hall, 1995.

Ballard, Carol. *Heart and Blood: Injury, Illness and Health.* Chicago: Heinemann Library (Reed Elsevier, Ltd.), 2003.

Gersh, Bernard J., Ed. *Mayo Clinic Heart Book.* New York: William Morrow and Company, 2000.

Gold, John Coopersmith. *Heart Disease.* Berkeley Heights, NJ: Enslow Publishers, 2000.

Gregson, Susan R. *Heart Disease.* Mankato, MN: LifeMatters, 2001.

Topol, Eric J., Ed. *Cleveland Clinic Heart Book.* New York: Hyperion, 2000.

Articles

Gorman, Christine, and Alice Park. "The Fires Within," *Time,* February 23, 2004, pp. 38–46.

Healy, Bernardine, M.D., et al. "Matters of the Heart: Special Report," *U.S. News & World Report,* December 1, 2003, pp. 37–70. (Series of nine articles.)

Langreth, Robert. "Attacking Heart Attacks," *Forbes,* June 21, 2004, pp. 152–165.

Underwood, Anne, and Jerry Adler. "What You Don't Know About Fat," *Newsweek,* August 23, 2004, pp. 40–47.

INDEX

Page numbers in *italics* refer to illustrations.

Low-density lipoproteins (LDL),
40–41, 83, 105

Magnetic resonance imaging (MRI)
scans, 59, *59*, 105
Medications, 65–67
MEF2A gene, 101
Mitral valve, 19, *20*
Mitral valve prolapse, 74–75, 106
Myocardial infarction, 26, 106
Myocardium, 106

Nicotine, 47, 86
Nitroglycerin, 65
Nuclear scanning, 57–58
Nuts, 82

Obesity, 12, 42–44, 87, 106
Omega-3 fats, 82, 100

Pacemaker tissue, 20, 34, 106
Pacemakers, artificial, 68–70, *69*, 70
Palpitations, 20, 106
Pericardium, 106
Physical examinations, regular, 52–54
PIA2 gene, 38
Pigs, and transplants, 95
Plaques, 23–25, 26, 49, 98–100, 106
Platelets, 106
Pulmonary circulation system, 14,
16, 106
Pulmonary valve, 19, *20*
Pulse, 18, 52, 106
Purple foxglove, 66–67

Radioisotopes, 57–58, 106
Rheumatic fever, 32–33, 106
Robotically assisted surgery, 99
Rubella, 32

Septum, 16, 34, 106
Sleep, 89
Smoking, 46–47, 86–87, 106
Spasms, 106
Sphygmomanometer, 52–53, 106
Stem-cell research, 96–98, 106

Stent, 70, 106
Stethoscope, 107
Stress, 48, 88–90
Stress test, *55*, 107
Stroke, 26–27, 66, 107
Surgery, open-heart, 71–75, *72, 73,
74*
Systemic circulation system, 14, 16,
107
Systolic pressure, 45, 107

Thrombus, 25, 107
Tobacco, smoking, 46–47
Trans fats, 79, 107
Transplants, heart, 22, 75–76, *76*,
94–95
Treatment
artificial pacemakers, 68–70, *69*,
70
balloon angioplasty, 70
heart transplants, 75–76, *76*
medications, 65–67
open-heart surgery, 71–75, *72, 73*,
74
Tricuspid valve, 19, *20*
Triglycerides, 41, 46, 107

U.S. Food Guide Pyramid, *81*, 81–83

Valves, heart, 19, 73–75, *74*, 105
Veins, 16, 107
Ventricles, 17, *17*, 20, 107
Ventricular fibrillation, 30, 107
Very low-density lipoproteins
(VLDL), 41

Weight, 77–78
White blood cells, 49
Withering, Dr. William, 66–67
Women
fatalities, 36
prevalence, 23
signs of heart disease in, 36

X-rays, chest, *56*
Xenotransplants, 94–95, 107